SOLDIERS
WITH
STAMMERING
VISION

DR ROBERT TYM
A/Prof Neurosurgeon then Psychiatrist

With a contribution from Psychologist
A/PROF BRENDON DELLAR

First Edition 2024
Copyright © Jeanette K P Tym
Published by Replete Press
info@repletepress.com

A catalog record for this book is available from the Australian National
Library and the British Library.

ISBN: 978-0-6486056-1-4 (Paperback)
ISBN: 978-0-6486056-2-1 (Hardcover)
ISBN: 978-0-6486056-0-7 (eBook)

THE FATHER OF CLINICAL OBSERVATIONAL MEDICINE
1624-1689

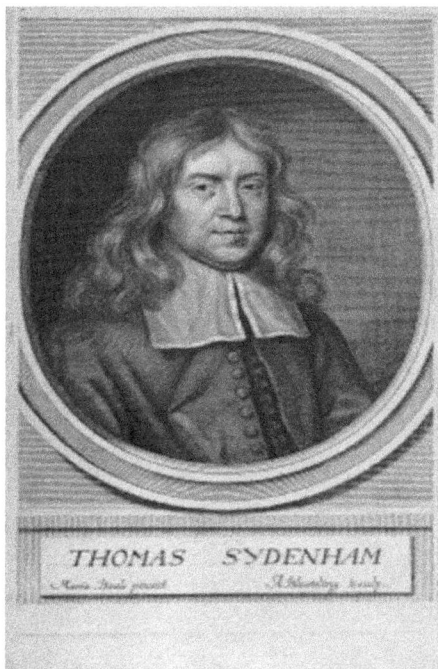

THOMAS SYDENHAM

**"Nothing in medicine is so insignificant
as not to merit attention."**

This is to remind us that a slow but better understanding of a serious anxiety disorder, PTSD— a disorder that can follow-for-life a person's experience of just one sudden surge of fear—arose from eventually ignoring a general reluctance to give any attention to an apparently insignificant 'something': the person's wavy vision.

A PRELIMINARY NOTE TO THE READER

This book is for everyone, but 'PTSD' is complicated. To make sense of it, we can't avoid having to use some 'technical' terms that may be new to the everyday person. The terms are fully explained in the context of the book and in the **Glossary of Terms.**

The **Extended Abstract** in Section One at the beginning of the book is for PTSD experts. It can be skipped over by the everyday person who can best start in Section Two, following the Glossary.

In the context of this book, **Post-Traumatic Stress Disorder ('stress' meaning only 'anxiety', a form of 'fear')** is defined as 'a mental disorder of anxiety,' and as understood by the common-sense language of everyday people: It is caused by, and follows at once or shortly after, a sudden experience of a mentally traumatic event (meaning a sudden anxiety-provoking or fear-provoking experience).

PTSD cannot be as presently defined in the Diagnostic and Statistical Manual of the American Psychiatric Association (the DSM) or in The International Classification of Disease of the World Health Organisation (the ICD), neither of which, as they are, make clinical or common sense to a clinician treating people with a PTSD.

THE BOOK IS IN TWO SECTIONS

SECTION 1

An extended abstract: 'what is newly understood about PTSD'

Mostly for the experts and others involved with PTSD.

SECTION 2 Part One
The Evidentiary Clinical Findings

For everyone interested in what PTSD is, how and from where the new evidence came, what can and can't be done about PTSD, and PTSD's place amongst common mental disorders and mental illnesses.

SECTION 2 Part Two
The Management of PTSD Type 1 and Type 2

Including the accurate diagnosis of PTSD with a simple visual test and how to properly perform EMDR (which cannot work for everyone, seemingly dependent mostly on their genes.)

DEDICATION

The book is dedicated to my grandfather, Walter Shepherd, who, in England on 12th December 1940, and to my grandson, Cyrus Fletcher, who, in Afghanistan on 2nd June 2009, were each killed by enemy action. They were both killed instantly by bombs, and without time to develop any PTSD. Also dedicated to all those over time who have developed PTSD, including my son, Ash, without whose expert help this book could not have been written. And dedicated not least, to my loyal wife and partner, Jeanette, without whose forgiveness and endless love and support there would certainly be no book.

ACKNOWLEDGEMENTS

John Llewelyn Burrell, LLB, Solicitor, who, in 1977, first drew my attention to several disabled compensation clients of his. They were suffering from a strange, unexplained, and disabling visual problem following mentally traumatic accidents at work. Being dissatisfied with the explanations of 'hysterical' and 'insignificant' given by various psychiatrists and ophthalmologists to whom he had referred his clients, asking for medico-legal reports, Burrell persuaded his clients' doctors to refer them to me, a psychiatrist who had previously been a neurosurgeon, and newly arrived in Australia. Burrell's medicolegal perspicacity, his disputing of the medical specialists' virtual dismissal of his clients' strange visual problems, had started the ball rolling for me. So, acknowledgement also to the many of my clients who co-operated in my clinical investigation of endless simple visual tests, and cooperatively maintained the impetus of my thirty-year-long exploratory clinical investigation into 'visual problems following mental trauma.'

CONTENTS

SECTION ONE 1

An Extended Abstract 3

For the mental health professionals and others wanting the new PTSD evidentiary clinical findings, and what can be reasonably inferred from them (without the long story of the finding of them).

Glossary 21

SECTION TWO: THE BOOK 25

For soldiers and first responders themselves and for everyone else wanting to know more of how uniquely complicated "PTSD" appears to be.

Introduction 27

Chapter One 35

Do the present-day 'authorised' definitions and descriptions of "PTSD" make any logical clinical sense? No, and why they were never meant to.

Chapter Two 51

A long-ignored subtle visual symptom, hinting at the possible neuro-biological nature of one form of "PTSD."

Chapter Three 61

What exactly is a 'persistently recurrent abnormal re-experiencing flashback memory recall'? And a note on Persistent Complex Bereavement Disorder.

Chapter Four 71

What exactly is the abnormal visual phenomenon 'persistent peripheral oscillopsia? (Plus: The independent evidentiary clinical findings of persistent peripheral oscillopsia.by Assistant Professor of Psychology, Dr Brendon Dellar.)

Chapter Five **85**

A clinical observational consequence: two different forms of PTSD: FORMAL DEFINITIONS of PTSD type 1 and PTSD type 2: the challenge to DSM and ICD.

Chapter Six **99**

A schoolteacher's account of his own PTSD type 1.

Chapter Seven **105**

The scientific experiment: transformational evidentiary clinical findings about PTSD type 1 and EMDR.

Chapter Eight **117**

The genomic-cum-neurobiology of PTSD type 1: two geneticists' most plausible and reasonable inferences from their personal evidentiary clinical findings.

Chapter Nine **133**

Finding ADHD and PTSD type 1 together more often than by chance.

PART TWO: SECTION TWO **143**

The management and treatment of PTSD type 1 and PTSD type 2.

Chapter Ten **145**

The simple but reliable, sensitive, and specific Visual Test for the presence or absence of PTSD type 1.

Chapter Eleven **151**

The simple and proper performance of EMDR trial treatment of PTSD type 1.

Chapter Twelve **157**

What treatments are best for PTSD type 1, PTSD type 2 and the personality disorder, Complex PTSD.

Chapter Thirteen **165**

Five different clinical cases of PTSD type 1 and PTSD type 2.

Chapter Fourteen **177**

PTSD type 1, ADHD, and Anorexia Nervosa all together—two different learn-from clinical vignettes.

Addendum **187**

What is a 'mental illness of depression', and what-and-why is ECT?

SECTION ONE

AN EXTENDED ABSTRACT

"PTSD" is a uniquely complicated disorder—virtually a 'Complex System'—with several interacting biological components, including genomic entities, two of which manifest as unique clinical symptoms. This abstract is written primarily for the 'experts'; it is not necessarily tailored for the everyday person, unlike Section Two of the book.

I am a retired psychiatrist, formerly an assistant professor neurosurgeon. During the first years of my clinical psychiatric practice, I initiated a prolonged exploratory clinical investigation. The investigation was *en passant,* lasting over a thirty-year-or-so period, into the neurological nature of an *obscure visual symptom—a visual abnormality*—that was being complained of by several of the first psychiatric patients referred to me. The patients with this *obscure visual symptom* were several immigrant women who had originally come to Australia from the Middle East and Southern Europe. Each of the several women had suffered frightening but not physically serious injuries at their various Australian work places some years previously, and through their lawyers, were each seeking workers' compensation. The women never met each other, but each woman was complaining of the same thing being present since their various accidents—a constant sense of wavy vision that seriously interfered with many things in their life and certainly with any attempt to return to work. Prior to being referred to me, they had each been referred—at the instigation of their lawyer—to either psychiatrists or ophthalmologists for medico-legal reports, and each woman had been independently diagnosed as 'hysterical', implying 'no physical injury to account for their visual difficulties, and compensation should be refused.' Their lawyer vigorously disagreed with the diagnoses of 'hysteria' being given to his clients. He had known them for over two or three years and trusted them. On hearing I had previously been a neurosurgeon, he came to see me and asked me to see each of them and give a second opinion on each of them. I saw each woman individually. I could not agree with the diagnosis of 'hysteria' either, but I had no other explanation.

Being somewhat nonplussed by this 'failure on my part', I decided that I must investigate this odd visual symptom seen in some psychiatric patients. To me, the symptom did not fit with the commonly seen 'hysteria'—a transient wavy vision that can accompany a transient panic attack or transient bursts of high anxiety. These women's symptoms had remained unchanged, persisting all day, every day, since the day of their accidents some years ago.

My exploratory clinical investigation started in 1977. Thirty years or so on, I had examined the vision of virtually every one of 9000 or so of my psychiatric patients for the same thing. Over the years, the investigation had merged into and ended as an investigation into the neurological nature of post-traumatic stress disorder, PTSD. I had first learned of the 1946 report of the 'stammering vision of the ex-soldiers from WWII with Traumatic Neurosis', mentioned on the Front cover of the book, when I was a third of the way through my investigation.

The clinical nature of this 30-year-long solo exploratory clinical investigation into any relationship between 'a specific visual abnormality and an experience of mental trauma', was aimed to satisfy The Standard 'Eight Guidelines of Scientific Methodology': viz, (i), The problem investigated was to be important; (ii), Prior knowledge was to be built on; (iii), There were to be no secrets; (iv), The design of the investigation was to be objective; (v), The final data was to be valid, reliable, and readily confirmable; (vi), The methods were to be simple; (vii), Any experimental data was to be fully testable-by-all and available to all; and (viii), Any inferences and practical applications taken from the findings had to be logical, had to be clinically predictable, and had to be clinically useful to all.

Hopefully, it will be seen from what follows that these eight guidelines above were adequately satisfied.

Firstly, and most importantly, the overall clinical observations—the accumulated evidentiary clinical findings—have contributed to the proof of concept of there being two superficially-look-alike but biologically different post-mental-trauma anxiety disorders, two distinctly different forms of what was called Traumatic Neurosis in 1889 by Oppenheim, two distinctly different forms of what was called PTSD in 1980 by the AMA and by The World Health in their ICD. As will be shown, (i), the two different disorders are con-generic, i.e. both disorders are caused by experiencing 'traumatic stress, but (ii), the two disorders are not conspecific, i.e. they are neurologically, genomically, and biologically very different from each other.

There have been many other anomalies, things unexpected, things in need of explanations, about PTSD, since the outset of my solo investigation I 1977. This book endeavours to provide some of those explanations in forms that are intuitively acceptable to most, if not to everyone. It all starts from the novel and readily-con-firmable-by-anyone evidentiary clinical findings coming from the exploratory clinical investigation into the hitherto ignored visual symptom. The symptom, it turned out, had 'first' (apparently first) been reported in the literature in 1946 as '*a stammering of perception in the periphery of the visual field*'. This was a symptom reported verbally by some ex-soldiers from WWII who were suffering from Traumatic Neurosis. This persisting symptom of 'stammering vision' was observed by and then reported by these ex-soldiers to the then-notable London ophthalmologist, Dr Harry Moss Tra-quair. Dr Traquair was carrying out routine examinations of the ex-soldiers' visual fields at the time. Dr Traquair was a nationally accepted expert on visual fields. He appears to be the first to report in the literature these subtle visual observations of the ex-soldiers—he reported them on page 121 of his short textbook*, but did so only very briefly, in just eleven words.

*Traquair, H.M., Introduction to Clinical Perimetry', 5th Edition, 1946,
London: Henry Kimpton. Page 121.

As far as we know, this observation of these ex-soldiers, if ever spoken of by others, was ignored by physicians other than Dr Traquair. When come across at all—it seems it was not deliberately looked for before, then, or since—it appears to have been routinely ignored in all branches of clinical medicine, including neurology, ophthalmology, and psychiatry. It was deemed a transient hysterical symptom, a symptom commonly complained of by very highly anxious people, especially in 'panicky people'—and 'best ignored', 'a symptom that isn't real', 'it goes away when they stop panicking', 'it's of no significance'.

When I had first come across the symptom in some of my psychiatric patients in 1977, I approached the most notable of my peers, the State's self-styled senior neuropsychiatrist, asking for a brief discussion on what was for me, a psychiatric beginner, a 'psychiatric visual mystery'. The phone response of this senior psychiatric peer was immediate and short: "No, thank you, doctor, I'd be embarrassed even to talk with you about it". I heard no more from him.

But Dr Traquair, in the 1940s, was examining the visual fields of people all day, every day. There is nothing about visual field testing, as it was then, to make anyone anxious at all, let alone very anxious. It seems only ex-soldiers with traumatic neurosis were reporting this 'stammering vision' to Dr Traquair when he was examining visual fields, and he thought it worthy of a mention in his textbook, if not worth any ophthalmological investigation.

The 'stammering vision in the periphery' is now called 'persistent peripheral oscillopsia', (osi-lop-sia), it is a Greek word for 'wavy vision'. Its clinical manifestations and the simple test for its presence or absence are given in detail below and throughout this book.

At a late stage of the investigation, in the early 2000s, well after Traumatic Neurosis had been re-named and re-classified as PTSD, and the use of EMDR treatment was being explored and found to be effective for some people with one of the two forms of PTSD (details coming later), I had briefly collaborated verbally with each of two patients who happened to be academic geneticists. The geneticists, who, as far as I knew, never met each other, had each been referred to me with one of the two forms of PTSD by their own but different doctors. Subsequently, both geneticists were totally cured of the same form of PTSD by the simple treatment technique of EMDR. I had been practicing EMDR treatment on that one form of PTSD ever since Dr Shapiro's paper appeared in 1989. (We come to EMDR at great length later)

Shapiro, F. (1989). Eye movement desensitization and reprocessing: A new treatment for posttraumatic stress disorder. Journal of Behaviour Therapy and Experimental Psychiatry, 20, 211-217. 989.

Over the time of their treatments with me, both geneticists became fully acquainted, verbally, with the evidentiary clinical find- ings of my exploratory investigations into PTSD. Both geneticists had been locally referred patients and were entitled to retain their anonymity. But each geneticist, willingly and independently, had conveyed to me their own most plausible and reasonable inferences taken from the clinical findings of their own clinical experiences, together with the evidentiary clinical findings up to that stage of the thirty-year exploratory investigation (as conveyed to them by me) on 'the nature of PTSD'. This follows the next paragraph.

The **body of this book** (in Section Two below) gives the history and details of the slow-coming-together of the evidentiary clinical findings over the 30 or so years of the exploratory clinical investigation. **This abstract** gives the readily-available-to-all evidentiary clinical findings of the investigation and the most plausible and reasonable inferences that can be taken from them, initially and most importantly, by the two geneticists and since then by others. The following inferences can most plausibly and reasonably be taken from the sum of the evidentiary clinical findings. **The full provenance of the evidentiary clinical findings is given in Section Two of the book.**

Firstly, there are two, and only two, forms of the anxiety disorder PTSD: there is a **PTSD type 1** and a **PTSD type 2**. The defining characteristics of the two are summarised in what immediately follows:

The defining characteristics of the *categorical* anxiety disorder PTSD type 1.

(The defining characteristics of the *dimensional* anxiety disorder, PTSD type 2, follow a few pages below.)

(i) PTSD type 1 is a ***categorical*** anxiety disorder. It is caused by, and only by, and at the moment of, an experience of a sudden surge of intense anxiety (fear, disgust), that, in some vulnerable persons, triggers an ***epigenetic insertion. An epigenetic insertion*** in this context is the tagging of a methyl group (CH3) onto some molecule of the DNA of a right-sided medial temporal gyrus integrated brain hub concerned with three separate brain functions: (a) with forming memory engrams, (b) with one aspect of the stability of visual focus of the oculo-vestibular reflex, and (iii) with the emotion of anxiety. This epigenetic insertion instantly perturbs the normal functioning of this integrated brain hub and instantly gives rise to the ***three abnormal clinical features of PTSD type 1***.

The first two of these three clinical features are unique to PTSD type 1—they appear in no other mental or physical disorder and are described immediately below. The third clinical feature, a persisting abnormally high level of anxiety and anxiety-related symptoms, is a generic symptom common to many anxiety disorders, including PTSD type 2 (see below).

(ii) One of the two *unique* features of PTSD type 1 is the recurrent memory recall of an ***abnormally formed memory engram***. On being recalled, the engram (the 'abnormal flashback of PTSD type 1') is recalled as an abnormal re-experiencing of (not just a normal account of) the noticed happenings and experiences ***during*** (i.e. contemporaneous with) the momentary sudden surge of high anxiety that triggered the epigenetic insertion. (The defining characteristics of *this unique form of recurrent abnormal flashing back memory engram recall* are described in more detail in the book.)

(iii) The second unique clinical feature of PTSD type 1 is **persistent peripheral oscillopsia**. The defining characteristics of this unique-in-form illusory visual phenomenon of movement of stationary objects are given in detail below and in the book. It occurs with the head and eyes held still and is distinct from the 'inconstant and disorganised' oscillopsia that can occur in transient high anxiety (panic); also distinct from the nystagmus-associated oscillopsia of Multiple Sclerosis, from other neurological disorders, and from the oscillopsia of peripheral vestibular disorders. It is believed to be the 'stammering of perception in the periphery of the visual field in Traumatic Neurosis' mentioned by Traquair in 1946.

(iv) The third clinical feature of PTSD type 1 is not unique; it is the **persisting, higher-than-normal-for-the-person level of anxiety and anxiety-related symptoms.**

(v) PTSD type 1 can be totally and permanently cured—but only in **some people** with PTSD type 1, **not in all people** with PTSD type 1—by the simple treatment technique discovered serendipitously in 1989 by psychologist Francine Shapiro. This treatment is called **Eye Movement Desensitisation & Reprocessing, (EMDR).** Properly performed EMDR—**but only in certain people with accurately diagnosed PTSD type 1, and only in people of certain phenotypes with PTSD type 1, not in people of all phenotypes with PTSD type 1**—can effect an **epigenetic reversal** in the affected integrated brain hub. In response to this de-tagging of the previously tagged DNA, the three abnormal symptoms pf PTSD type 1 go—they go together, step-by-step and in-step—and the patient is fully and permanently cured of ('one module of', see later below) their PTSD type 1.

(vi) It appears clinically that among those people most likely to be cured of PTSD type 1 by properly performed EMDR are of the phenotype light coloured eyes, fair skin, and fair hair. It appears clinically that among those people least likely to be cured of PTSD type 1 with EMDR are those of the phenotype dark eyes, dark hair, and olive skin. (There is no explanation for this other than to say that genotype plays some part in the overall construct of PTSD type 1.)

(vii) For those people with PTSD type 1 who are unaffected by properly performed EMDR, i.e. those whose genome appears to prevent EMDR from being effective, their PTSD type 1 persists lifelong. Their anxiety can be greatly and permanently assuaged by Exposure Therapy, but their two PTSD type 1 'unique' symptoms persist, albeit with a diminished anxiety level and obtrusiveness.

(viii) For those people who are of the phenotype ADHD impairments, there appears to be a very increased risk for them to develop PTSD type 1 in response to experiencing a sudden surge of intense anxiety. Their risk appears to be significantly higher than it is for those who are not of the phenotype ADHD impairments.

(ix) PTSD type 1 has not been seen to occur in those under five or six years old. However, those who are five or six years or older and accurately diagnosed with PTSD type 1 have the same chance as older individuals with PTSD type 1 of successfully responding curatively to properly performed EMDR treatment. Children under the age 5 years who are of the phenotype ADHD will have the same chance as all other genotypes of experiencing mental trauma in the form of a sudden surge of extreme anxiety—and if they develop an epigenetic insertion in response, then they *might* develop some other form of mental disorder, e.g.., some form of autism spectrum disorder—we don't know.

("Fifty to 70 percent of individuals with ASD have ADHD. Adults with ASD are more than four times more likely to be diagnosed with PTSD (type 1 most probably) than adults without ASD." NIH.)

(**x**) PTSD type 1 can have been caused by an experience of an event of **any degree of objective** severity, from mild to severe. PTSD type 1 has a spectrum of **any degree of subjective severity**, from mild to severe.

(**xi**) People can develop more than one **module of PTSD type 1** in response to experiencing more than one sudden surge of intense anxiety. **Each module, with its own unique abnormal flashback with its own persistent peripheral oscillopsia and its own raised anxiety,** requires its individual successful EMDR treatment for the person to be totally rid of their PTSD type 1.

(**xii**) **The diagnosis of PTSD type 1**. Since persistent peripheral oscillopsia is unique to PTSD type 1, then a simple visual test for the presence or absence of persistent peripheral oscillopsia (a simple test described in detail below and in the book) proves to be a sensitive, reliable, and specific test for the presence or absence of at least one module of PTSD type 1, regardless of what other mental or physical disorder is present at the same time: *but with the exceptions* of blindness, of severe permanent oscillopsia from some other diagnosable neurological disorder, or of the person's uncooperativeness. The Visual Test takes thirty seconds to perform, requires no apparatus, hence costs nothing, and is applicable to anyone over the age of five or six years.

(xiii) What we can infer from the evidentiary clinical findings of the neurobiological nature of successful and unsuccessful EMDR treatment of *one module* of PTSD type 1.

EMDR treatment involves: (i), The memory evocation of the recurrent abnormal re-experiencing memory engram of one module of the person's PTSD type 1. (ii), Having the person hold that memory evocation while simultaneously conducting a run of full bilateral saccades at one to three per second, and continuing the run of full saccades until the evoked abnormal memory engram involuntarily fades from the person's awareness. (iii), The same runs of full saccades are repeated—until no tiniest fragment of abnormal memory engram can be evoked, despite trying, and that abnormal form of memory engram is fully replaced by a normal-in-form memory engram of an account (no longer a re-experience) of what had been noticed and remembered during the moment of the surge of intense anxiety that initiated that module of the person's PTSD type 1. (iv), If there was only one module of PTSD type 1, then a repeat Visual Test will show a total absence of persistent peripheral oscillopsia. (v), If the person has no other source of significant anxiety, then there will be a relative absence of the anxiety and anxiety-related symptoms that had been present at the time of the recurrent abnormal re-experiencing memory engram, or any fragment of the anxiety that had been evoked during the initial runs of saccades.

In short, during successful EMDR, there had been a step-by-step and in-step diminution and finally, elimination of the three abnormal symptoms—the abnormally high anxiety, the abnormal form of memory engram, and the abnormal form of peripheral vision: that final module of PTSD type 1 has been permanently eliminated.

(xiv) What we can infer from the evidentiary clinical findings of the neurobiological and genomic nature of the effect of properly performed EMDR on a module of properly diagnosed PTSD type 1.

Most reported regional cerebral blood flow studies in "PTSD" have shown a preponderance of increased blood flow in the region of **the right** temporal gyrus and the amygdala nucleus rather than the left. Magneto-encephalogram studies report increased electro-activity in the temporal regions of the brain of those with "PTSD" but no differential right-left localisation in the temporal regions of the brain.

It is most plausible and reasonable to infer that the 'integrated nodal brain hub 'location' of the neurological abnormality of PTSD type 1 is an 'integrated nodal brain hub' located in the right-sided medial temporal gyrus. The medial temporal gyrus is a bilateral site common to (i), the juxta-positioned amygdala nucleus subserving memory formation and storage, (ii), the 'centres' for anxiety (fear) and disgust, and (iii), the oculo-vestibular nucleus, which subserves the oculo-vestibular reflex. This reflex involves normal reflex bilateral eye saccades in response to normal head movement—whilst the eyes are focussed on some stationary object and the head moves to one side, the eyes reflexively saccade to the opposite side to maintain their focus prior to the head movement. And, if the eyes saccade in response to a new visual stimulus, the head reflexively moves in the same direction accordingly.

EMDR consists of bilateral saccades with the head stationary and in the presence of (i), a surge of abnormally high anxiety from the abnormal re-experiencing engram, and (ii) the evoked epigenetic (CH3) tagged DNA molecule of the abnormally formed memory engram. Intuitively, during the saccades of EMDR, one can envisage some form of perturbation of the affected right-sided brain hub that effects an epigenetic reversal—but only if the person's genome permits it. This removal of the (CH3) tagging allows the completion of, or a correction of, the abnormally formed memory engram to a normally formed memory engram of the happenings noticed during the experience of the momentary event of a sudden surge of high anxiety.

If the 'macro-physicality' (at the molecular level) of a single epigenetic insertion, a single methylation tagging of a methyl (CH3) group to some DNA molecule, had caused the PTSD type 1, then it is reasonable to intuit that that insertion of physical information—a physical methyl group—would have to be unilateral, either in the right temporal area or the left temporal area, not in left and right simultaneously. The corpus callosum, the thick band of nerve fibres arching over the third ventricle to connect the right and left cerebral hemispheres, ensures, presumably, that the 'micro-physicality' (at the quantum level) information that one hemisphere possesses is also shared with the other hemisphere. In PTSD type 1, blood flow studies suggest it is the right-sided temporal gyrus where the molecular epigenetic insertion has taken place and where successful EMDR effects the demethylating epigenetic reversal. (Perhaps sadly, we have made no note of any effect that handedness may appear to have on any clinical manifestation of PTSD type 1 or PTSD type 2.).

The diagnostic *visual illusion* (the Visual Test) of persistent peripheral oscillopsia does not involve saccades, but if the test is positive, the *illusion of oscillation* is of the *expected effect* that rapid saccades would require to keep focus on the illusory side-to-side movement of stationary objects in the periphery of the visual field if the peripheral objects were moving from side-to-side in reality.

The high anxiety of a panic attack or near panic can alone, without PTSD type 1 or PTSD type 2 being present, produce transient and irregular illusions of stationary objects seen throughout the whole visual field to be moving about irregularly, and not just confined to the periphery of the visual field. Hence, a stipulation when conducting the Visual Test for persistent peripheral oscillopsia is that the Test cannot be performed until a panic attack or near panic has completely subsided. So, as always, clinical practice benefits from clinical practice.

A module of PTSD type 1 can be fully responsive to, i.e. can be fully and permanently eliminated by, EMDR *within the first few seconds of the first saccades of EMDR treatment,* or its elimination may take many half-hour sessions of runs of saccades repeated over days, weeks, or months before the module is fully eliminated. We note again that PTSD type 1 takes no more than a second or two to fully develop and that, exceptionally, PTSD type 1 *can, but not always does, take* no more than a second or two to be fully eliminated. (Information Theory suggests one must treasure one's exceptions— exceptions carry more information than the usual.) Epigenetic mechanisms are the only mechanisms that can effect such dramatic changes in the brain so quickly, as the two geneticists pointed out.

As judged by the constantly increased blood supply in the region of this right-sided brain hub in PTSD type 1, this brain hub remains in a constant hyper-energetic state. Presumably, this per- sistent extra energy is required to persistently maintain, all day, all night, year in, year out, the details of the abnormal memory engram of the event, the persistently higher than necessary anxiety, and the persistent peripheral oscillopsia. If this was due to a hyper-energetic surge of high anxiety triggering a hyper-energetic epigenetic inser- tion into some DNA—some DNA concerned with mature memory engram formation—then this hyper-energetic-unstable state can be overcome by the mechanism of EMDR acting on this brain hub. But only if the person's genome permits this return to the lower-en- ergetic state that entropy is expecting it to return to.

What we do not know about PTSD type 1.

We do not know, cannot intuit, the mechanism for the involvement of the person's genotype in determining the likelihood or otherwise of the person developing PTSD type 1 in response to experiencing a sudden surge of anxiety, or, of determining the likelihood or oth- erwise of the person with PTSD type 1 responding successfully to properly performed EMDR.

What we need to know.

How to effect an epigenetic reversal in those with PTSD type 1 whose genome will not permit EMDR to be effective. **And what we must not forget to do** is arrange effective exposure therapy for those with

PTSD type 1 for whom EMDR cannot be effective and do the same for those with PTSD type 2.

PTSD type 1 has not been diagnosed in those under the age of five years. Perhaps it cannot have been diagnosed because of a lack of childhood memory formation (so-called childhood amnesia) and PTSD type 1 is not there, But: it is not known if experiences of sudden mental shock in those under five years of age or so, especially those who have the genome for ADHD impairments, can suffer from other types of brain damage and other mental disorders from mental-trauma-related epigenetic insertions, e.g., some forms of autism-spectrum-like disorder.

Knowing what we do know about PTSD type 1, more research with Genome-Wide Association Studies, with functional brain imaging together with successful EMDR treatment for PTSD type 1, might contribute new and clinically helpful insights into PTSD type 1.

The defining characteristics of PTSD type 2.

If a person does not (perhaps cannot—their genome won't allow it to happen) develop PTSD type 1 in response to the experience of a sudden surge of intense anxiety, or, a person experiences a less sudden mentally traumatic event, then the person may develop the **dimensional** anxiety disorder PTSD type 2.

While PTSD type 1 is a unique **categorical** anxiety disorder, having two unique clinical features not present in any other mental or physical disorder, PTSD type 2 is a generic **dimensional** anxiety disorder, having no unique clinical features, just having persisting higher than-normal-for-that-person anxiety, with one or more anxiety-related symptoms that always include a distressing but normal-in-form memory of the causal event. The anxiety-related symptoms can be much the same as those that can be present in the anxiety disorder PTSD type 1, hence the 'superficial' clinical similarity between the two biologically different anxiety disorders, PTSD type 1 and PTSD type 2, that can follow mental trauma.

There have been no evidentiary clinical findings to suggest that either a person's genes or a person's age influences any clinical characteristic, including response to treatment, of PTSD type 2.

The distressing-to-recall memory engrams of PTSD type 2 are accounts of objective, mental, and emotional experiences and **not of abnormal-in-form re-living or re-experiencing** the frightening and distressing events. **Properly performed EMDR treatment has no effect on the distressing normal-in-form memories of PTSD type 2.** A person may have many modules of PTSD type 2 from many different mentally traumatic experiences.

A person may have **both** PTSD type 1 and PTSD type 2 together, arising from one experience of a mentally traumatic event or arising from two or more different mentally traumatic events at different times. If a person with both PTSD type 1 and type 2 is cured of PTSD type 1 by EMDR, then PTSD type 2 is left to be treated separately.

PTSD type 2 can resolve spontaneously over time but not always does, depending on its severity and or on a persisting mentally traumatic later-life environment.

The definitive treatment for PTSD type 2, as it is for EMDR treatment-resistant PTSD type 1, is exposure therapy, usually with the aid of anti-anxiety medication or other anxiety-relieving substances—perhaps CBD or MDMA or similar, taken under psychotherapeutic supervision.

When 'EMDR' is done for wrong reasons, done wrongly, and done for long periods, then it might be acting as exposure therapy for unpleasant memories that are related or unrelated to PTSD type 1 and or PTSD type 2 and claimed as a success for 'EMDR'—ignoring the presence or absence of persistent peripheral oscillopsia.

So-called Complex PTSD.

This is not a third type of PTSD. It is, in effect, a distressing personality disorder due to the long persistence of inescapable severe mental trauma that, over time, damages the developing or developed personality. There may be several modules of PTSD type 1 and or PTSD type 2 mixed in.

Its defining characteristics can be similar to those of 'Borderline Personality Disorder plus PTSD'. Treatment requires efforts to get rid of both forms of PTSD, together with long-term supportive psychotherapy, possibly exposure therapy and non-addictive anxiety-relieving medication.

Formal clinical definitions of the anxiety disorders PTSD type 1 and PTSD type 2.

These are postulated to be suitable for inclusion in a Diagnostic Manual of Mental Disorders and an International Classification of Mental Diseases. They are given in Section Two, Chapter Five, of the book.

The details of the Visual Test for the presence or absence of PTSD type 1.

The simple Visual Test is a sensitive, reliable, and specific test for the presence or absence of persistent peripheral oscillopsia, unique to PTSD type 1. Hence, it is a sensitive, reliable, and specific test for the presence or absence of PTSD type 1, regardless of the presence of any other mental or physical disorder (other than blindness or frank uncooperativeness).

Without the routine and simple use of The Visual Test, there will be many with the anxiety disorder PTSD type 1, of any level of severity, left un-noticed and untreated. (Full details of The Visual Test are in Section Two, Chapter Ten. Full details of the simple proper performance of EMDR treatment for PTSD type 1 are in Section Two, Chapter Eleven.)

Figure One. The simple Visual Test. How the examiner performing the test appears to the right eye of the person being tested during the Visual Test. Note that the tip of the examiner's fingers reaches the periphery of the right visual field exactly. The examiner must adjust his distance from the person being examined to ensure this is the case.

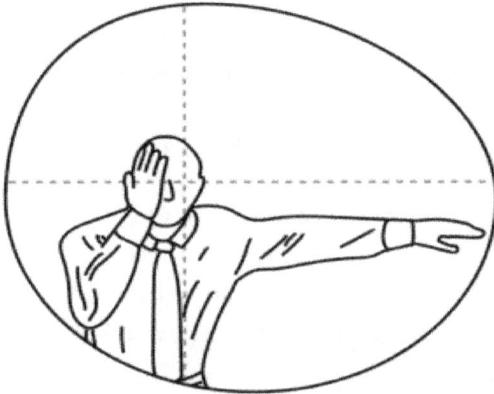

Picture by Silas Tym

The person being tested is sitting a meter or so away. They have their left eye covered, and their right eye is fixated on the pupil of the left eye of the examiner. The examiner has the right eye covered. The oval is the outline of the right visual field of the person being tested. The centre of the crossed lines is the visual axis held rigid between the pupil of the left eye of the examiner and the pupil of the right eye of the person being tested. This mutual fixation ensures that during the ten seconds of the test, the person being tested does not momentarily blink or shift the fixation of their right eye off the examiner's left eye unnoticed by the examiner. The mutual fixation lasts for ten seconds. At the end of the ten seconds, the person being tested is asked to demonstrate with their right arm how the examiner's left arm had appeared to them during the ten seconds.

Postscript to the Abstract.

The smart German neurologist Hermann Oppenheim, in his 1898 book, 'Die Traumatischen Neurosen' (Traumatic Neurosis), had envisaged, ". . . some form of physical consequence to fright, a molecular tissue change, some real and tangible damage to the brain, of those with what others are referring to as 'hysteria following injury' . . .". Today, Oppenheim, with the evidentiary clinical evidence regarding 'PTSD type 1, and its successful EMDR treatment, appears to have been amazingly prescient: an epigenetic insertion and its epigenetic reversal is certainly intuitively 'tangible damage'.

Post Traumatic Blast Disorder (PTBD)

When an experience of a mentally traumatic event is in the form of the exposure to an explosion and its blast wave - the propagation of a supersonic pressure gradient - then the impact of this is a blunt head injury, a Traumatic Brain Injury (a TBI), whether or not the experience also causes a PTSD type 1 and or a PTSD type 2. This TBI can be of any severity---with blast wave-related compressions and shearings of the brain tissues -giving micro- and macro-brain haemorrhages, and diffuse brain nerve cell axon injuries, all with short or long-term diverse effects, each virtually recoverable or virtually irrevocable.

With experiences of multiple blasts - gunshots, bomb blasts, shell blasts (whether the person is at the sending or receiving end) the long-term effects can be that of any oft-repeated TBIs (seen in boxers, contact field sport players, even in late-age brain atrophy) i.e., a widened third ventricle seen on brain imaging. Combat veterans and bombed-out civilians, with the double diagnosis of PTSD type 1 and or PTSD type 2 plus PTBD, are probably most noticeable *en masse* in combat veterans and collateral refugees. There is no specific active treatment for Post Traumatic Blast Disorder, PTBD (except in extreme cases of brain swelling where induced coma in a specialised unit may be used).

GLOSSARY

Categorical Clinical Disorder. A unique clinical entity, having one or more characterising features that are unique (meaning, features not found in any other mental or physical disorder) and are also invariant (meaning, they are unchanging). The disorder can be of any level of severity. The disorder can be present with other disorders. PTSD type 1 is a categorical clinical disorder (as are Chicken Pox, Huntington's disease . . . but not PTSD type 2.)

Cognitive dissonance. A feeling of emotional discomfort from having to believe in two different things it is believed cannot both be right. It is a cognitive dissonance that can hinder one's judgement in assessing the veracity of apparently conflicting new evidence.

Complex PTSD. The name given to the clinical features of a dimensional personality disorder engendered by the experiences of long-term mental trauma from having long-term or constantly repeated and or persisting PTSD type 1, PTSD type 2 and or other mental trauma.

Counter-intuitive. Contrary to what most people would presume was common sense. **Intuition**. Based on what one feels to be true even without conscious reasoning; instinctive.

Dimensional Clinical Disorder. A disorder characterised by a variable cluster of some non-unique clinical features. The disorder can be of any degree of severity. It can be present with other disorders. PTSD type 2 is a dimensional disorder, an anxiety disorder caused by one or more experiences of mental trauma.

EMDR. Eye Movement Desensitization and Reprocessing. A simple technique of combining rapid side-to-side eye movements (called saccades) while holding in the mind an abnormal form of just one flashing-back memory recall of PTSD type 1. Properly performed, EMDR can only cure some, not all, people with PTSD type 1, and cannot cure any other mental or physical disorders. It cannot cure PTSD type 2. (See Epigenetic Reversal)

Engram. An engram is a hypothetical change in the brain that accounts for the existence of a memory—of the happenings during a circumscribed moment in time or of an object or fact.

Epigenomics (Epigenetics) Changes caused by a modification of gene expression (a modification of what the gene normally does in the body) that can be environmentally induced.

Epigenomic (Epigenetic) insertion. The insertion of a chemical group, usually a methyl group (CH3), that tags onto a DNA molecule, a gene, and thereby modifying the gene's function. An epigenomic change in this context (PTSD type 1) is triggered by the experience of a sudden surge of intense anxiety, a 'mental shock'. PTSD type 1 cannot be inherited by the next generation. In some but not all with PTSD type 1 there can be an epigenomic (epigenetic) reversal when the methyl group is de-tagged from the molecule, and the normal functioning of the gene is restored, and PTSD type 1 is cured. (See EMDR).

Evidentiary Clinical Findings. Clinical findings relating to or affording clinical evidence. Clinical findings of evidentiary value.

Generic Disorders. Defining characteristics of or relating to a class or group of similar disorders with no unique features; for example, most anxiety disorders, non-psychotic depressive disorders, personality disorders have generic features. PTSD type 2, aside from its association with mental trauma and the presence of disturbing memories of that trauma, has the anxiety symptom features of a generic anxiety disorder.

Genome. The genome of an organism is the whole of its hereditary information encoded in its DNA molecules, its RNA, and its proteins.

Genotype. The unique genomic constitution of a particular individual.

Genomics (Genetics). The branch of molecular biology concerned with the structure, function, evolution, and mapping of genomes,

Intuition, to intuit (see Counter-Intuitive, above)

Mental Disorder. A long persisting mental state characterised by personal distress and impairment in multiple areas of life.

Intuitive. Having the ability to know or understand things without any proof or evidence.

Mental Shock. A sudden surge of intense anxiety triggered by a sudden and unexpected experience of fear and or disgust, triggered by experiencing a sudden and unexpected mentally traumatic event.

Module of PTSD type 1. The unique and invariant 'compound double-symptom' that completely characterises PTSD type 1: i.e. 'a symptom of a persisting abnormally formed memory engram of what was experienced during a moment of mental shock', that is invariantly linked to the symptom of 'persisting peripheral oscillopsia'. Subsequent experiences of a sudden surge of anxiety from experiencing subsequent mentally traumatic events, can give rise to more modules of PTSD type 1, giving a multi-modular PTSD type 1.

Oscillopsia. Pronounced 'osi-lop-sia'. A Greek word for 'wavy vision'. There are several forms of oscillopsia associated with different forms of neurological and vestibular system disorders.

Persistent peripheral oscillopsia. A form of oscillopsia unique to PTSD type 1. A persisting illusory appearance of oscillation of stationary objects seen in the periphery of the visual field when the eyes are kept focussed on a stationary object ahead. This is colloquially known as 'wavy vision in the periphery' and once called 'a stammering of perception in the periphery of the visual field'.

Phenotype. The set of certain recognisable characteristics of an individual or group of individuals, e.g., 'their skin colour', 'their eye colour', 'their hair colour', 'their having ADHD'.

Stammering Vision. An unofficial and imprecise name once given in 1946 by an ophthalmologist to a form of 'wavy vision' in the periphery of the visual fields being reported to him by some ex-soldiers from WWII with Traumatic Neurosis. See 'persistent peripheral oscillopsia' above.

Trauma (a noun) meaning damage, physical or functional.

Traumatic (an adjective) meaning damaging.

Traumatic Neurosis. The name given to post-traumatic stress ('stress' meaning anxiety) disorder by the German neurologist Professor Hermann Oppenheim in 1898. The name was changed to PTSD in 1980 by the American Psychiatric Association. (The terms 'shell shock', 'battle fatigue', etc. were common war time and after-the-war slang terms for the same disorder).

Visual Test for PTSD type 1. A simple, reliable, specific, and sensitive test for the presence or absence of persistent peripheral oscillopsia, and hence for the presence or absence of PTSD type 1.

SECTION TWO: THE BOOK

INTRODUCTION

THE SOLDIERS WITH STAMMERING VISION

In the early 1900s, Dr William Osler, the man still known to all of us as The Father of Modern Medicine, and one of the founders of Johns Hopkins Hospital in Baltimore, reminded all physicians for all time: "Medicine is a science of uncertainty and an art of probability." In this book, we are limited to initially collecting evidentiary clinical findings from a thirty-year-long exploratory clinical investigation and, secondarily, creating a series of most probable and reasonable inferences from those findings on what has gone wrong inside the brain in PTSD—as certain as we can be and hopefully as most probable.

This book, about new information on the nature of PTSD, is written for the everyday person and for the mental health expert alike—an expert being anyone involved with anyone, including themselves, who has PTSD. The book starts and finishes with the significance of a simple, accidental re-discovery of a long-ignored, subtle, and *unique visual symptom* of PTSD. This visual symptom was reported by some ex-soldiers from WWII who had Traumatic Neurosis (the previous name for PTSD). This visual symptom was called, at that time, 'a stammering of perception in the periphery of the visual field'. Each of those ex-soldiers had reported this visual oddity to an eye doctor who was examining their visual fields at the time. The eye doctor, a prominent London ophthalmologist, Dr William Ross Traquair, had written of this odd visual observation reported to him by these soldiers in the book he was writing on visual fields. It was Dr Traquair, a Scotsman, not the soldiers, who called it a 'stammering vision'. He wrote his book in 1946. It *appears* to be the first ever mention of this visual symptom with Traumatic Neurosis.

The mention of it in Dr Traquair's book *appears* to have been left ignored for seventy years. Presumably, this subtle visual symptom (this simple clinical observation reported only by some ex-soldiers and recorded in only eleven words in Dr Traquair's small textbook) was thought too simple, too insignificant a symptom to warrant any attention. Indeed, even in recent times, it has been thought too insignificant to warrant the attention of the majority of psychiatrists, psychologists, ophthalmologists, and 'PTSD experts' alike—they all *appearing* to think the idea that it could be significant was clinically nonsensical.

But, this odd 'bit' of new information, the observations of those soldiers of a unique visual symptom associated with their Traumatic Neurosis, has turned out to be the lynchpin of a new understanding of PTSD. The evidence for this new understanding has come from a thirty-year-long exploratory clinical investigation into visual abnormalities associated with mental trauma. This new understanding of PTSD gives us the most plausible explanation of the epigenomic, genomic and neurobiological nature of there being two forms of post-traumatic stress disorder. One form of PTSD does have this subtle, simple symptom of vision; the other form of PTSD does not have this subtle, simple visual symptom.

So, we must conclude, from the evidentiary clinical evidence we shall come to, that there must have always been two forms of what PTSD was called in the past: two forms of Traumatic Neurosis, two forms of 'Shellshock', two forms of 'Battle Fatigue'; and now, two distinct forms of today's PTSD. The 'stammering vision in the periphery of their visual field', has been present in all those with one of the two forms of PTSD, and never in those with only the other form of PTSD.

Arising from this, as the evidence shows, it transpires that there is one form of post-traumatic stress disorder from which people can never recover spontaneously over time, the form of PTSD that has 'stammering vision in the periphery of the visual field', and there is the other form of PTSD from which people can recover spontaneously over time, and that form of PTSD has no stammering vison in the periphery of their visual field. So, PTSD, by whatever other name it has been given over time, PTSD has always been significantly misunderstood by us all.

When the American Psychiatric Association (APA) published its new Diagnostic and Statistical Manual of Nervous Diseases in 1980, the section on Post Traumatic Stress Disorder did not, and still does not today, make clinical commonsense to the mind of the treating clinical psychiatrist or psychologist, and certainly not to a patient. The same still goes for the section on PTSD in the International Classification of Diseases, the ICD, of the World Health Organization, the WHO.

For reasons of clarity, and from the outset, this book defines 'PTSD' simply and sufficiently as 'an anxiety disorder caused by one or more experiences of frightening and or disgusting mental trauma, and PTSD can come in two different forms, as a PTSD type 1 and or as a PTSD type 2'.

This book describes the slow evolution of the new evidentiary clinical findings that have come from the thirty-year exploratory clinical investigation and describes what can most reasonably and plausibly be inferred from those new evidentiary clinical findings. This book then answers the following big questions about "PTSD":

What are the two forms of PTSD, actually? What has gone wrong inside the brain in one or the other of the two different PTSDs? What can be done about the PTSDs? And now, how, and why can properly performed EMDR treatment permanently cure some people with a PTSD type 1 and not everyone with a PTSD type 1, and EMDR cannot help anyone with a PTSD type 2 or with any other mental or physical disorder? And what is so special about EMDR? How and why might it work? And why can some people with a PTSD type 2 recover spontaneously over time? Why can people with a PTSD type 1 never recover spontaneously? Is there a reason why some people are more likely than others to get a PTSD type 1 and why some other people get a PTSD type 2?

In addition, how some people get PTSD type 1 or PTSD type 2 after experiencing a subjectively terrible mental trauma and some people, in the spectrum of objective severity, get one or other after experiencing an objectively trivial mental trauma. And how some people get PTSD type 1 and or PTSD type 2 very severely, in a spectrum of subjective severity, and some people get one or other or both very mildly. We don't know, but we strongly suspect that some people cannot get PTSD type 1 and can only get PTSD type 2.

These answers are the inferences regarding the many clinical, epigenomic, genomic, and neurobiological observations of the many people who can recover spontaneously from PTSD type 2, of the many people who can never recover spontaneously from PTSD type 1, of those who cannot recover spontaneously from PTSD type 1 but can recover completely with properly performed EMDR treatment, and of those who cannot recover spontaneously from PTSD type 1 and can never be cured by properly performed EMDR treatment.

That there must be two different PTSDs, a PTSD type 1 and a PTSD type 2, is 'lexical semantics', i.e. a want of simplicity to still comply with the philosophical dictum known as Ockham's Razor: "Explanations that postulate fewer entities, or fewer kinds of entities, are to be preferred to explanations that postulate more". The evidentiary clinical findings tell us there must be two forms and only two forms of PTSD, not just one. (So-called Complex PTSD, which we come to later, cannot be a third form of 'PTSD'—it is a form of personality disorder caused by having one or both forms of severe 'PTSD' over a long period, interfering with the developing or developed personality).

In 1889, the German neurologist, Herman Oppenheim, conjectured that the cause of what we now call PTSD type 1 was "some molecular change in the brain caused by a fright" to explain what he had named "Traumatic Neurosis". The concept of anything being 'epigenetic' anywhere, which we come to later, only became possible after Conrad Waddington, the great Cambridge, UK geneticist, coined the term in 1942. At the time, it was not thought it had anything to do with any Traumatic Neurosis. It was only in 1946 that the London ophthalmologist Dr Harry Moss Traquair wrote of the observations of those ex-soldiers with traumatic neurosis having: "a stammering of perception in the periphery of the visual fields in ex-soldiers from WWII with Traumatic Neurosis." It was only in 1977 that this author, this psychiatrist, embarked on his solo 30-year exploratory investigation into a unique abnormal visual symptom reported to him by several of his patients, knowing nothing at that time of Dr Traquair's previous findings. It was only in 1980 that the American Psychiatric Association re-formulated Traumatic Neurosis into PTSD. It was only in 1989 that the American psychologist Dr Francine Shapiro reported her clinical observation of EMDR being 'a cure for PTSD'. It was only in 2009 that two senior geneticists, each having experienced PTSD type 1, and its cure by EMDR, plausibly and reasonably inferred an epigenetic insertion as a most reasonable and plausible conjecture for Oppenheim's "molecular change in the brain", and an epigenetic reversal for Dr Francine Shapiro's EMDR 'cure for PTSD'.

A question that may well be asked by anyone at this stage: Are these conjectures, or inferences drawn from the clinical evidence, true? The only possible answer is: No scientific endeavour can ever claim to finally solve any complex scientific problem; the best that anyone can strive for, PTSD included, is 'a new truth-for-today', a provisional better understanding, a 'fresh understanding for today, based on reasonable and most plausible inferences taken from the newly available evidentiary clinical findings': a more rational and more useful understanding of 'PTSD' than the past understandings, one that yields fresh clinical benefits of diagnosis and treatment for the people with 'PTSD', and (hopefully) opening new paths for new genomics research into new much-needed cures for those whose PTSD type 1 will not respond to EMDR.

Any new truth-for-today is always contingent and open to scrutiny and dispute by anyone at any future time. Every 'truth' can start off as a heresy and just might end up as accepted orthodoxy for a time: only time tells. People might want to know why there have been no multiple reasonable and plausible inferences about 'PTSD', just this one? Well, so far, there are few, if any, geneticists investigating 'PTSD types 1 and 2', and few, if any, psychiatrists or psychologists investigating the genomics of PTSD type 1. One must wait for fresh clinical or other evidentiary clinical findings from which conflicting inferences can be drawn.

So, scepticism is always welcome, but scepticism cannot come together with a refusal to test out the new evidentiary clinical findings, regardless of how counter to one's intuition the clinical findings and inferences drawn from them might initially appear. There is no shortage of people with PTSD with whom this simple evidence given in this book can be simply but thoroughly tested.

The re-discovery, the 'new' evidentiary clinical findings, have come from novel clinical observations, from the ex-soldiers from WWII, and from Dr Shapiro's walk in the park. They have not come from any attempt at present-day 'classical research', not come from one or more people setting out to try to solve a problem about 'PTSD'. There was no application for a research grant, and no ethical or other sanctioning ethical committee to satisfy—and there was a refusal for help from Research Gaters, who said that my overall project was not 'real research'. The initial curiosity, leading over time to the 30-year-long exploratory clinical investigation, was the observation of a perspicacious compensation lawyer, who reported his observations to me in 1977. My serendipitous encounter with this lawyer is told in the text of the book. The serendipitous arrival of two patients, both academic geneticists, both with PTSD, clinched the 're-discovery'.

In 2009, the bare clinical essence of the new evidentiary clinical findings of the investigation, and some of their implications, was written up anecdotally by me and two occasional clinical associates: a senior ophthalmologist and a senior neuropsychologist. The manuscript was peer-reviewed and published in the international, part-psychiatric, part-psychological journal, Traumatology.

1 Tym, B., Beaumont, P., Lioulios, T. *Two Persisting Pathophysiological Visual Phenomena following Psychological Trauma and their Elimination with Rapid Eye Movements: A Possible Refinement of Construct PTSD and Its Visual State Marker. Traumatology. 15(3): 22-33 (2009).*

It is one thing to find something new, surprising, and counter-intuitive, quite another to get the new information out to those whom one might think would benefit from knowing of it, let alone to get them to believe it. To date, thirteen years later, the peer-reviewed paper has been cited only 15 times.

The contents of this new book is not rocket science either, but simple clinical science, clinical observations, evidentiary clinical findings from talking to, examining, and following up 9000 or so different people, and the logical, plausible, and reasonable inferences taken from the clinical findings. Nothing terribly clever; hopefully, clinically beneficial to anyone over five or six years old and living anywhere and unlucky enough to be stuck with a post-traumatic stress disorder.

The book aims to be suitably Mertonian in terms of the Sociology of Science. Here are Merton's three demands in this description of something new about PTSD —hopefully something that's more than a 'just-so-story':

Universalism. Scientific claims must be held to objective and preestablished impersonal criteria. Such a value can be inferred by the scientific method.

Communality. The findings of science are common property to the community, and scientific progress relies on open communication and sharing.

Disinterestedness. Science should limit the influence of bias as much as possible.

Organised Scepticism. The necessity of proof or verification that subjects the field of science to more scrutiny than any other field.

These points stress the value of the easy reproducibility of the evidentiary clinical findings upon which the book mostly rests.

CHAPTER ONE

Do the present-day 'authorised' definitions and descriptions of 'PTSD' make any logical clinical sense? No, and why they were never meant to.

Recent progress in understanding more about PTSD has thrived on serendipity, scattered observations, bits of information, accidental clinical findings, mostly coming in from 'left field', some seemingly trivial, but all finally, and luckily, joining up. In 1946, the London, UK, ophthalmologist Harry Moss Traquair was examining the visual fields of some ex-soldiers from WWII with Traumatic Neurosis from WWII. His ophthalmological super-speciality was mapping visual fields. Each eye has its own visual field, meaning the total that *one eye* can see when kept still and focussed on a point straight ahead. The total visual field is the entirety of what can be seen with *both eyes* open, kept still, and focussed on the same point.

Two-thirds of the human brain is concerned with vision one way or another. Damage to different parts of that two-thirds of the brain can affect the visual fields in different characteristic ways; hence Traquair, from mapping the visual fields, could map sites of localised brain damage, if any. He was examining the soldiers' visual fields in the way visual fields were always examined in 1946. We do not know exactly why he was examining them. Presumably, he was looking for evidence of physical brain damage that might help explain something about Traumatic Neurosis.

What Traquair did find was unexpected and inexplicable: an abnormal visual phenomenon in ex-soldiers with Traumatic Neurosis, but not present in people without Traumatic Neurosis. How did this come about? During the standard visual field test, those soldiers, like all others who were being tested at the time, were told to keep their head and eyes perfectly still, to close one eye, and with the other eye focus steadily on a stationary black dot in the middle of a visual field chart held directly in front. While staring at the black dot—not glancing away from it even momentarily—they were told to take notice of what was happening in the outer ring of their visual field, around the periphery of their vision. Dr Traquair would slowly move different small, coloured discs from outside their visual field into the perimeter of their visual field, and, as he did so, the soldiers were to report to him as soon as they saw the discs coming into their field of vision. There is nothing about a visual field test to make anyone anxious. Oddly, each of the soldiers with Traumatic Neurosis also reported to Dr Traquair that after a few seconds of staring with one eye at the black dot, all the stationary objects they were aware of in the periphery, the outer perimeter of their vision, including the coloured discs that were being moved in, appeared to start moving, waving about, going up and down or going side to side. This wavy vision of stationary objects only in the periphery of their visual field persisted until they looked away from the black dot, and it then stopped immediately. It started again after a few seconds of staring at the black dot again. It happened with either eye. Nothing to be anxious about. Traquair did visual field testing every day and virtually all day. He wrote books on it. He tested the visual fields of many people with different brain and eye conditions, not just soldiers. Apparently, only ex-soldiers with Traumatic Neurosis volunteered to him their observations that things seemed to move about in the periphery of their visual field during the visual field test. Traquair must have thought the soldiers' observations to be significant exceptions to what is usual. Apparently, no one without Traumatic Neurosis ever mentioned it to him while their visual fields were being tested. Traquair paid sufficient attention to this visual oddity that he mentioned it in his later 1946 textbook on 'Visual Fields', albeit in only eleven words, and left it at that. '**A stammering of perception in the periphery of the visual fields**' in the soldiers with Traumatic Neurosis. The word 'stammering' means a 'rhythm perception'. Traquair, being a Scot, might well have said a 'choogling' of perception, but it means much the same thing to a Scot: a rhythm and an undulation. Thomas Sydenham, the Father of Observational Medicine—his portrait is the Frontispiece of the book—would have been pleased that he did mention it in his book. There is no evidence that Traquair investigated it, or thought it to be of any great significance, but he did take the trouble to mention it and pay it a bit of attention. Perhaps he thought someone might be interested one day. He had nothing else to say about the visual fields of soldiers with Traumatic Neurosis, as far as we know.

One day in 1986, while perusing the basement library of the Sydney Eye Hospital, I came across Traquair's book* by chance, forty years after it had been written, and nine or ten years after I had started my own investigation into the same abnormal visual phenomenon, a visual phenomenon that Traquair had called 'stammering vision'.

*Traquair, H.M., Introduction to Clinical Perimetry', 5th Edition, 1946, London: Henry Kimpton. Page 121.

One must presume that Traquair thought his observation of the soldiers' observations was an exception. Perhaps Traquair was aware of the maxim to which all investigators are told to abide, doctors included: "Treasure your exceptions". This maxim is now part of modern information theory: 'Unusual events and experiences carry more information than common events and experiences.' Traquair's bit of serendipity has turned out to be a tiny bit of new 'truth' about human vision, and a big bit of new 'truth' about PTSD seventy or so years later. So far as is known, this discovery of Traquair's, recorded in the form of a brief mention of this wavy vision of soldiers with Traumatic Neurosis, was ignored, presumably deemed insignificant by others, if taken notice of at all. It was certainly insignificant to the soldiers. Perhaps they only noticed it when they were at the ophthalmologist's office having their visual fields tested, and Dr Traquair did not appear to do or say anything about it anyway. They most probably forgot all about it themselves—they were unlikely to forget their Traumatic Neurosis, their PTSD type 1 that would be with them for the rest of their lives.

Most of the words in this book end up being about those eleven words of Traquair's. Presumably, those ex-soldiers had not taken notice of this wavy vision in the periphery of their vision before because, like the rest of us, they never spent much time staring with one eye at a black dot for minutes on end. Had they looked to see what was waving about in the periphery during the visual field test, they would have immediately seen there was nothing waving about. If the rest of us sense something moving at all in the periphery of our vision, then we instinctively and immediately turn our heads and eyes to see what it is. If there is nothing to be seen, we ignore it. All mammals and many other animals do the same, their visual systems attuned to be vigilant for unexpected movement anywhere, especially in the periphery. Nonetheless, these likely-to-be-very-vigilant soldiers had reported their own observations: what they experienced when they stared with one eye straight ahead for some time and saw things moving out of the corner of their eye and were not allowed to move their head and eyes to see what, if anything, was moving. On a battlefield and seeing movement in the periphery of the visual field, they would instinctively look, perhaps see an enemy sniper, and be just in time to save their lives, shooting the enemy sniper first.

Observations are facts. Facts are best seen without the distortions of prejudice. When many separate people report the same observations, the facts become more believable, 'more credible facts' and more worthy of attention being paid to them by others. At the time, whatever the unknown significance of these particular facts might be, they were not totally ignored by Traquair. That was a bit of serendipity, 'a happy accidental finding'. This was thirty-four years before the name Traumatic Neurosis was changed to the name PTSD. Today, visual fields are tested quite differently, with no chance of anyone noticing wavy vision in the periphery of the visual field if any wavy vision is there.

There had been more serendipity, another happy accidental finding, in 1977. This was three years before the name Traumatic Neurosis was changed to PTSD. A compensation lawyer, a lawyer whose job it was to legally represent disabled workers in the Worker's Compensation Court, clients disabled due to injury at work, was mystified by the disabilities complained of by several of his women clients. Several women had separately engaged him and engaged him at different times over the previous two to three years. The lawyer's legal firm specialised in Workers Compensation and had many clients who were immigrants from many different countries. These several women clients of the lawyer were all immigrants from the Middle East and Southern Europe. They didn't know each other; they never even met each other. But each was seeking individual help from the lawyer for their long-persisting disabilities following their various frightening and traumatising accidents at their separate workplaces. In addition to their aches and pains left over from their various not-all-that-severe accidents, they were all reporting, complaining of, much the same thing: a very peculiar persisting visual problem that left them unable to see properly. They each reported the same observation, the same fact: that everything they looked at appeared to be 'waving about' all the time, not just now and then, not just when they were staring. This abnormal visual symptom, they all reported, dated from the time of their accidents two or three years previously and the same symptoms were not going away. None had suffered any head or eye injuries in their accidents, and none of their accidents was very physically serious. They had all been somewhat frightened by their accidents, not surprisingly, but not injured physically in any serious way. They had all continued to be frightened, anxious, and unable to return to work since their accidents. The lawyer knew all about the usual work injuries but knew nothing about this exceptional and obscure visual complaint of these several women from the Middle East and southern Europe.

As usual, the lawyer had referred these women to medical specialists—psychiatrists and ophthalmologists—asking them for medico-legal reports for him to present to the Compensation Court on his clients' behalf. Much to the lawyer's consternation, each of his clients had been diagnosed by these various specialists as being 'hysterical'. This implied that in the specialists' opinions, there was nothing physically wrong to find with their bodies or their eyes or their brains, so the symptoms had to be related to their anxiousness, and at this late stage, their anxiousness had nothing to do with their accidents several years ago. 'False' or 'illusory' physical symptoms, due solely to anxiety, were then, and still are called by many, 'hysterical symptoms', 'nothing physically real'.

To the mind of this perspicacious lawyer, however, the consensus of these local ophthalmologists and psychiatrists diagnosing 'hysteria' in these several different women, women all with much the same long-standing and stable visual symptom, appeared wrong to him, intuitively wrong. True, being relatively new migrants, all the women were anxious about not being able to work. Being a new migrant in any country predisposes one to anxiousness about fitting into new ways of doing things, new customs, and languages to understand, let alone earn a living to house and feed their family. These clients could not return to work because of a mixture of their anxiety and their wavy vision. They were no longer able to support their families financially. They hoped for compensation. Their lawyer believed they were entitled to compensation. To the specialists who had examined them, seeing them for a limited amount of time, not seeing more than one of them each, it had seemed reasonable to think such a person to be grossly exaggerating, consciously or subconsciously, their inability to return to work in the hope they could get compensation to live on, and not have to go back to factory work. Presumably, they were not thought to be *consciously* malingering, deliberately lying about their visual symptoms. Being hysterical implied to the specialists that they were *unconsciously* exaggerating, and, once they had their compensation, if awarded, their anxiety would go away, and they would recover from their aches and pains and quickly regain their proper, stable eyesight. Many other lawyers and specialists around town at the time even suspected there were some half-organised conspiracies amongst immigrant groups seeking worker's compensation for spurious made-up symptoms. Some small number of immigrants, as well as non-immigrants, were caught out being *untruthful* about their disabilities. This lawyer intuitively sensed that these several women he had been seeing over several years, did not fit the mould of 'migrants with hysterical symptoms spuriously seeking compensation for wavy vision'. There was something 'genuinely' wrong with them.

But it is certainly well known by many everyday people, not just physicians, that when anyone suddenly becomes acutely anxious, perhaps someone with a panic disorder, and at the height of a panic attack, they may well complain of having inexplicable wildly-wavy-vision. Some saying, ". . . help, everything looks to be swaying, waving about . . . it's making me feel dizzy. . .". This illusory wavy vision settles back to normal stable vision ten minutes or so later, when the acute anxiety lessens. The various names given for this particular *transient* visual oddity, and to other odd and inexplicable *transient* pseudo-physical neurological symptoms in people who are very anxious, vary between 'somatising symptoms', 'functional symptoms', 'conversion disorder symptoms', all symptoms 'explained' by 'the person's brain, somehow or other, subconsciously converting anxiety into a body-like, a somatoform, experience, perhaps for some reason such as drawing attention to their anxiety, or perhaps for 'no reason'. There is plenty of well-known clinical evidence to suggest that high anxiety can trigger many forms of odd symptoms for which there is no explanation other than 'somatising', 'functional', 'conversion'. These new words are there merely to replace the old word, 'hysterical'. Hysterical was Hippocrates' word for the same clinical phenomena centuries ago. All four of those words are meant to mean 'imaginary, not real, no physical abnormality, nothing medical for doctors to worry about, the symptoms will go away'. The diverse clinical features of functional, somatisation and hysteria had never been explained neurobiologically, so no one knew how to explain what anxiety is doing to the nervous system, triggering seemingly 'false' clinical symptoms that go away on their own. Perhaps they are subconsciously concocted 'red herrings' 'functional neurological disorders' (FNDs), including 'functional seizures'. Giving a name, 'hysteria' or 'somatising', or 'FND' to replace a clinical explanation, then stating that the name *is* the explanation, is best called circular reasoning. This is hardly surprising when all the bizarre somatoform, functional, hysterical symptoms eventually *do* disappear on their own when the anxiety goes. The person is no worse off for having had them. The symptoms are soon forgotten about, with nothing left to explain. In the end, they are clinically insignificant for the person and are safely ignored by the doctor, so perhaps it doesn't matter what name they're given. Malingering, 'consciously, deliberately, pretending to be ill in order to escape duty or work' is an auxiliary explanation for inexplicable somatoform symptoms. It is a dangerous diagnosis to make, a diagnosis that can be mostly right, but just occasionally can be proved wrong, making the diagnostician look foolish and arrogant. However, the 'wavy vision' of these lawyer's clients, clients from the Middle East and Southern Europe, wasn't going away over time.

But a big but: there is now some good evidence, evidence we knew nothing of in 1977, that the association between 'high levels of anxiety' and 'illusory 'wavy vision' does have a neuroanatomical correlate—a 'non-hysterical' genuine explanation. Much later in the book, we come to the close neuroanatomical association, in the region of the amygdala nucleus, a closeness between an anatomical 'source of anxiety production', and an anatomical source of 'illusory perception of movement in the visual field' in the adjacent part of the oculo-vestibular reflex system. The insular cortex of the brain, deep inside the lateral sulcus of the cerebral hemispheres, appears to be a site of an 'integrative brain hub. 'Brain hubs' link large-scale brain systems; they are 'multimodal integration sites', which is 'how the brain is said to work'. We come back to these highly significant anatomical facts in Chapters Four and Eight, where we have to find an explanation for the actions and non-actions of EMDR treatment.

Long-persisting high anxiety itself certainly can give rise to life-shortening genuine physical disorders. Sudden high anxiety certainly can give rise to sudden lethal heart attacks from Takotsubo cardiomyopathy—sudden death from sudden grief. High anxiety can give rise to an increase in 'stress hormones' secreted from the adrenal gland, hormones that can be measured. Anxiety can do a lot of other things, suddenly or over time, in many ways that cannot be measured.

The lawyer knew these several women with 'stammering vision' well. He thought intuitively that the specialists' medical reports written about them were simplistic, not really making any *common* sense. It seemed to him that it was more than coincidence that these women had virtually identical presentations, and all came from similar parts of the world, Southern Europe, and the Middle East. They had symptoms that he, the lawyer, had not been told of by his Northern European clients, his more usual clientele. The women appeared ingenuous, straightforward, honest people. The lawyer could not see how all the clients could be purposely 'hysterical' in the same way, and about their vision, and consistently so for so long, for the two or so years he had been seeing them and trying to help them.

Any idea that it could be explained by their 'culture', that is 'the ideas, customs, and social behaviour of a particular people or society', could not make any intuitive common sense to their lawyer either. He had seen them together with their children and with their husbands when they had been accompanied by them to legal consultations. His legal firm was not making any extra money out of continuing to see them. He felt he needed some medical person from somewhere to give their symptoms 'proper attention': to explain the visual complaints, and write sensible medical reports for him to take to court. He would have to represent them all individually in the Workers' Compensation Court sooner or later.

The lawyer, on hearing ". . . there is a new psychiatrist in town; he used to be a neurosurgeon . . .", decided he would visit me personally, discuss his dilemma over these women, and ask if I would see them, give an opinion, and write sensible medico-legal reports on them.

I was at the outset of my psychiatric career. I had left neurosurgery, and after spending four years re-training to become a psychiatrist at the Institute of Psychiatry in London, UK, I was setting up my own solo clinical psychiatric practice in this new country. I was in no position to refuse to see them. At that stage, in 1977, I knew very little about Traumatic Neurosis and nothing about Dr Traquair. I did not come across that book and taken notice of any eleven words on page 121 until nine years later, in 1986.

I saw the women one at a time over a week or so. No ex-neurosurgeon could ignore any visual symptom. Here were several women, all reporting the same visual symptom, the same observation, persisting wavy vision everywhere they looked. Having seen these several women in consultation, each separately over two or three weeks, I agreed with the lawyer: I did not know what was causing their persisting visual disturbance, but a diagnosis of 'hysterical' did not make any intuitive or other clinical sense to me either. My neurosurgical and neurological experiences were mostly among northern European populations, so perhaps it was not surprising that I had never come across the likes of this symptom before if it was only a common symptom in the Middle Eastern and Southern European ethnic communities.

Once again, clinical observations are facts. All clinical observations merit attention to some degree. When several people report the same clinical observation, bizarre and counterintuitive as it might seem, the fact becomes more credible. Credible, exceptional facts certainly merit more attention. Such facts, and clinical findings, may or may not turn out to be clinically significant. But each of the previous specialists, psychiatrists, and ophthalmologists had only seen one each of the women. Hearing one seemingly bizarre observation spoken of by only one woman would have less impact than hearing several identical seemingly bizarre observations spoken of by several different women who had never met each other but all of an uncommon-for-Australia-at-the-time ethnicity.

In the consultations with me, all the women had much the same story to tell, and all told of much the same observation. Their wavy vision was there all the time and everywhere they looked, whether their head and eyes were still or they were walking around and looking around. They could not ignore it. The visual symptom seemed genuinely neurological, not transiently somatoform. It begged an explanation. The lawyer's intuitive hunch seemed reasonable. This persisting oddity of vision was a *clinical exception* for me as it was for the lawyer. The scientific maxim said *treasure your exceptions* and it applies to everyone and to information theory in general.

This triple-word maxim or gnomic, *treasure your exceptions*, originated from the constant theme of a controversial biologist and geneticist, the late-nineteenth to early-twentieth-century man from Yorkshire, William Bateson. Based on certain aspects of some of his own *exceptional* biological findings, Bateson argued endlessly with Charles Darwin over the validity of aspects of Darwin's overall theory of evolution based only on Darwin's biological findings. (In that context, Bateson's theme may soon be vindicated by recent exceptional biological findings in epigenetics and computational biological modelling, theories of evolution that are becoming daily, hourly, more complicated.)

I was powerless to do anything about the plight of these several women, unable to help them, never having seen the likes: disabling wavy vision of that nature persisting unchanged for years on end, and no abnormal neurological or ophthalmological physical finding to account for it. These women certainly had anxiety disorders following physically trivial but frightening-to-them accidents. One woman from slipping from an ordinary workbench stool and merely bruising her buttock. All the women had been treated for years by their various doctors with various anti-anxiety and anti-depressant medications. They had all been counselled by those who understood them, their culture, their religion, and their language. Medication and talking therapy had been of no help to them. It was 1977; there was no name for PTSD, just Traumatic Neurosis, with the word neurosis sounding much like the word neurotic, not far from sounding rather like the word hysterical in the minds of many everyday people. In 1977, when these women were seen, the name for a long-persisting disorder of pain and anxiety following very frightening experiences was Traumatic Neurosis, also called Shell Shock or Battle Fatigue. These women did not seem to fit any of those names. One of the women, having slipped from a stool while working at a factory bench, was hardly the most terrifying of experiences in the eyes of most people knowing anything about soldiers' Traumatic Neurosis and Shell Shock.

In 1980, Traumatic Neurosis was reformulated by the American Psychiatric Association, the APA, and the name changed to Post Traumatic Stress Disorder. This reformulation was not to define a newly specified clinical disorder *per se,* but to find a way of fairly compensating military personnel from the Vietnam War suffering from Traumatic Neurosis. The Veterans Associations needed a way of differentiating those, amongst the many ex-service personnel suffering varying degrees of disabling and persisting anxiety and flashing back memories who could claim compensation, distinguish them from those less affected who, the VA thought could not, should not, claim compensation. As with those from WWI with severe Traumatic Neurosis, not all could be compensated. In Germany following WW1, there was no money left for any ex-soldiers with Traumatic Neurosis to be compensated.

So, those Vietnam Veterans, men and women, whose history

and clinical examination results fell *below* certain thresholds of the severity of objective war-related causes, and below certain thresholds of subjective clinical symptoms, were not to be given a diagnosis of PTSD, but were to be given varying other diagnoses such as Adjustment Disorder, and they were not to be given compensation.

This left the diagnosis of PTSD and the availability of compensation being restricted to those who had experienced *only certain specified* frightening events, not just any other equally frightening events, and who had *only certain specified* severe anxiety symptoms, not just any equally severe anxiety symptoms. What the *causes* had to be, and what the *symptoms* had to be for the diagnosis of PTSD were strictly specified in the APA's Diagnostic and Statistical Manual of Mental Disorders, the DSM.

So, PTSD, according to the APA and the Dept. of Veteran Affairs, was not to be, could not be, a *discrete clinical entity*, could not be a discrete mental disorder, categorical or dimensional. Only if one had what the APA and the Veteran Affairs Board said one needed to have to get the 'diagnosis', i.e. the 'label', PTSD, then could one get compensation. No matter how severe the cause was, and no matter how severe the symptoms were, if they didn't 'fit', then one didn't have 'PTSD'. This clinical nonsense suited the staff of Veteran Affairs, who were not doctors, and who could now administer the available funds for compensation more easily. It left the world's psychologists and psychiatrists confused and frustrated, and a lot of others confused and frustrated. But all this is explicable by PTSD turning out to be so unexpectedly complicated.

So, as good as the DSM is for everything else, their version of PTSD has to be ignored, and the same with the version of PTSD in the World Health Organisation's International Classification of Diseases.

The subjective severity of the symptoms and the objective severity of the accidents of these women with wavy vision who are being described here, would certainly not have fitted the criteria for PTSD. Nowhere in the DSM, or in the WHO's ICD that had copied the clinically confusing DSM criteria for PTSD, was any mention made of any persisting visual symptoms being associated with PTSD or with any form of mental trauma or mental disorder.

These several women with wavy vision duly went to court to fight for their due, some *compensation* for their work-accident-related persisting disability, with their hopes pinned on me, 'the new psychiatrist' giving the 'expert evidence of a doctor' on their behalf. But each woman was returning home with the predictable verdict: 'no compensation for hysteria'. The presiding judges preferred the 'expert evidence' of the experienced ophthalmologists and psychiatrists of the defence to that of the Johnny-come-lately psychiatrist from Yorkshire, England, for the plaintiff saying he didn't know but couldn't agree with his peers that it wasn't 'real', that it was 'hysterical'. Subsequently, these women were followed up for some years to see what became of them. I remained powerless to help them. None improved in any way. They were eventually lost to my follow-up. In retrospect, I called them 'The Ladies with Stammering Vision'.

Given the laws of probability and several exceptional observations of a strange and persisting visual oddity, I had little option other than to see if it did have any clinical significance, and if so, what. Having seen these women, I assumed I would be seeing others with the same in my future clinical practice. I decided to look further for any clinical evidence of persisting visual oddities of persisting wavy vision in other people with psychiatric-cum-psychological disorders, following trauma or not following trauma. I was curious and didn't want to be caught out in the future.

The official clinical name for disorders of wavy vision is 'oscillopsia', pronounced *'osi-lop-sia'*, a Greek word for wavy vision. The name oscillopsia is rarely, if ever, mentioned together with the so-called 'hysteria' of wavy vision associated with high levels of anxiety during a panic attack.

There are several different forms of oscillopsia and several different ophthalmological, neurological, and inner ear disorders that cause the different forms of oscillopsia. I had worked in an Institute of Neurology, together with a neuro-ophthalmologist from an Institute of Ophthalmology; I had worked as an Assistant Professor of Neurosurgery, including working in northern Europe, southern Africa, and North America—but never in southern Europe or the Middle East. I was well acquainted with the several different ophthalmological, neurological, and inner ear disorders that could cause oscillopsia. Those women did not have oscillopsia as listed or depicted in any of the textbooks on ophthalmology, neurology, or otology.

On re-visiting my academic psychiatric mentors, the London psychiatric cognoscenti, a few years later, seeking their advice on this oddity of vision, I was just short of being told: ". . . the 'wavy vision' is hysterical . . ." and was told ". . . psychiatric patients say a lot of funny things ...". These were the joint considered responses of an academic neuropsychiatrist and an academic psychologist at an internationally acclaimed academic institute. I had no option but to investigate this 'wavy vision' myself as far as I could investigate it. I would be fostering 'cognitive disequilibrium' if any new clinical information were to contradict the acquired beliefs of my learned psychiatric, neurological, and ophthalmological peers and mentors.

CHAPTER TWO

A long-ignored subtle visual symptom, hinting at the possible neuro-biological nature of one form of 'PTSD'.

There was nothing special about my taking up the investigation. Any other psychiatrist with a neurosurgical or neurological background and presented with the same unusual coalescence of clinical circumstances and the women with 'wavy vision', would have done the same. Chance coalescence of unusual circumstances always presents challenges to the curiosity of anyone. I would be seeing a lot of people with psychological and psychiatric problems in my forthcoming psychiatric career. The people I would be seeing would be of all ages over five or six to eighty, from all walks of life and of many different ethnicities, though mostly northern European. I could not be selective about whom I saw; anyone could be randomly referred to me by many different doctors. Fees were never to be an issue; only those who could easily pay, paid; the others were covered by the country's near-universal healthcare. I would be practicing in several different regions of South-eastern Australia. I would be seeing people in my office and some in the hospital where I had admitted them. I would be following them up, and they could be following me up to complain should things go awry. I was not to be a 'remote' academic psychiatrist, overseeing junior psychiatrists in training—the only ones closely involved with people with psychiatric disorders, and only for a short time in academia. Some of the people would be returning to see me on and off for over thirty to forty years.

It would not take up much time in any psychiatric consultation to ask a few brief questions about vision. It was an obvious routine in neurosurgery to ask about vision. This adjunctive clinical investigation would have to be exploratory, with no idea where it would lead if it were to lead anywhere. It would be heuristic, 'learning as you go', an investigation of collecting observations and collecting thoughts. I had a friendly and co-operative, initially sceptical, ophthalmologist and a friendly and co-operative, initially sceptical, clinical neuropsychologist to call on for help and advice: in the end, both eagerly contributed to the publication of the scientific paper on the findings published in the psychiatric literature in 2009. We will come to the publication of this paper later. I would be asking each person referred to me, briefly, a few simple questions about their vision, particularly about any experiences of 'wavy vision', and briefly ask about their experiences of frightening accidents, frightening experiences, in the past. The questions would be leading questions asked, regardless of the reasons for the persons' referrals to me as a psychiatrist. I would also be asking anyone who was not referred, anyone who would agree to answer the same questions, including my own relatives, friends, and the friendly office cleaners.

Over time, there were people who, when specifically asked, said they did have or had had experiences of one or the other or both: 'wavy vision' and or seriously frightening experiences in the past. Those people were, in the early years, few and far between. Some people, when asked, and said they did have experiences of very significant and frightening accidents at some time in the past, and also said they had unwanted anxiety symptoms stemming from the time of the frightening experiences. And some of those people, but not all of them, said they had experiences of' wavy vision' but some said they had never had any. Some who had noticed 'wavy vision' said it had been only when they were extremely anxious, almost panicking. Some others said their 'wavy vision' was only after they were staring at something for more than a moment or two, and it went away when they looked away, so they took no notice of it. An ex-soldier said his 'wavy vision' was while driving at night with his eyes steadily focussed on the yellow line in the middle of the road: the yellow line would quickly appear to be wobbling side to side, and it would stop waving about only when he momentarily looked away but would come back again after a few more seconds of concentrating on the yellow line. He said that he did have 'flashbacks' of a frightening event, but said he was not going to talk about those.

For many, not all with any sort of 'wavy vision', it was noticed only out in the periphery of their vision and after a few seconds of staring. One or two said their 'wavy vision' was all over their whole visual field when they stared at anything for too long. Very few said their 'wavy vision' was of any significant trouble to them.

If enough people were to be seen to make sense of what it was all about, then the investigation would have to go on for a long time. People referred to any psychiatrist have many diverse problems. Many of the people referred had one or other of the many different types of anxiety disorder. Only with hindsight did all these early reports of peoples' observations make any clinical sense—some reports of 'wavy vision' and experiences of frightening moments in the past, and some reports of experiences of frightening moments in the past but no reports of wavy vision.

After the first year or so of the investigation, a simple eye test was devised to detect any 'wavy vision' if it were there. A very simple Visual Test, a test as 'fool-proof' a 'subjective test' as possible, taking all of 30 seconds to perform. A simple Visual Test that has no apparatus, so it costs nothing to perform. A simple Visual Test, but it is a test that has turned out to be sensitive, reliable, and specific to detect the presence or absence of this form of 'wavy *vision' that is present when steady gaze of one eye is maintained for up to 10 seconds on a stationary object.* The simple test is described in detail in Chapters Four and Ten, (see Figure One). The test simply ensures that a person being tested does not move the steady gaze of their eye away from a stationary object held at the centre of their vision — their eye does not move undetected one tiny bit for the whole ten seconds of the test. After ten seconds of steady gaze, the person being examined is asked to demonstrate how they saw a particular stationary object in the periphery of their vision appear to move if it did appear to move. Anyone can learn to perform the simple Visual Test and perform it on anyone who is over five or six years old — the exceptions being a person who is blind or a person who is uncooperative.

This form of 'wavy vision' in the periphery of vision had to be given a name; it was called Persistent Peripheral Oscillopsia, (pronounced *osi-lop-sia,* a Greek name for 'wavy vision'). Persistent Peripheral Oscillopsia is explained in detail in Chapter Four. It is called 'persistent', because if it appears during the simple Visual Test at some time in the ten seconds of staring, then it *always, persistently, appears at that same time during the ten seconds of any subsequent Visual Test for that person.* If steady gaze is maintained for more than ten seconds, then it is seen to persist until steady gaze ends. It is called 'peripheral' since (for most people that I was seeing with it at that time) the oscillopsia (the wavy vision) was confined to the periphery of their visual field.

The oscillopsia in those women I first saw — the women from Southern Europe and the Middle East — all had their oscillopsia over the whole of their visual fields and the oscillopsia was there all the time, with no delay in appearing. It became apparent that the persistent peripheral oscillopsia, when present, varied in its severity and extent over the visual field depending on the person's ethnicity.

Once the test had been devised — not exactly difficult to devise — every person being referred was asked to participate in the simple test. Thirty seconds of visual testing did not take up much of the ninety minutes of any psychiatric consultation time. The clients might or might not have thought me, the psychiatrist, a bit eccentric — I was careful not to explain what the Visual Test was testing for before the test was performed. Other psychiatrists who heard about it certainly thought this psychiatrist was eccentric — and readily dispensed the usual *ad hominem* reserved for colleagues deemed to be eccentric, non-conformist, and possibly 'clinically unsafe'.

Some people with persistent peripheral oscillopsia were asked to see my ophthalmology colleague. He checked their vision as he checked any other person's vision routinely. No other visual abnormalities or explanations were found to explain it. Just three of those people with persistent peripheral oscillopsia, and checked by the ophthalmologist, also agreed to a further investigation at the Visual System Research Unit. This investigation was to exclude persistent peripheral oscillopsia being accounted for by the normal 'micro-saccades'. 'Saccades' is the name given for rapid side-to-side eye movements, movements of scanning to-and-fro between two fixed points, one at the extreme left and one at the extreme right. Micro-saccades are normal and totally unnoticeable by oneself; tiny, tiny, very rapid, side-to-side scanning eye movements are always present on a normal, steady gaze. They prevent the retinal cells of the eye from over-exposure to steady light during steady gaze, or at any time when the eyes are open. This investigation from this research unit showed to their satisfaction that micro-saccades, as detected by movements of a sensitive infra-red beam shone onto the eyeball, were not synchronized with the persons' apparent sensations of wavy vision movements of objects in the periphery. Micro-saccades could not be an explanation for persistent peripheral oscillopsia.

Three of those people with persistent peripheral oscillopsia were investigated at the Vestibular Disorders Research Unit to exclude their wavy vision being accounted for by any *abnormality of their balance mechanisms in their midbrain or inner ear.* No eye, ear, or neurological disorder was detected to explain the persistent peripheral oscillopsia; there was only the 'wavy vision'. The *cause,* the pathological neurobiology of persistent peripheral oscillopsia, was left unexplained at that stage of the overall investigation. *The cause of Persistent Peripheral Oscillopsia is most reasonably and plausibly inferred by the two geneticists we come to later in Chapter Eight.*

As the 30 or so years of the investigation slowly progressed, this 'few people' with this form of oscillopsia and a history of frightening experiences became a few hundred people out of the nine thousand or so people who were eventually seen and examined. The nine thousand people who had been seen were of all walks of life and all ages over five or six years old. They were seen in a country, southeast Australia, with a mostly northern European population. There were people of many other ethnicities in that population. Some of the people seen, of southern European and Iberian ethnicities, had much more pronounced oscillopsia, and many were all too well aware of it before being asked and tested. One person from southern Italy had persisting and troublesome oscillopsia over her whole visual field, the same as that of those several women from the Middle East and Southern Europe who were seen initially; the women referred to me originally by the lawyer, the women with 'stammering vision', who had triggered the investigation in the beginning. (The clinical case, the vignette of a person from Southern Europe, is described in more detail in Chapter Thirteen, Case 3.)

The investigation had been ongoing for three years when Traumatic Neurosis was reformulated by the American Psychiatric Association and branded to Post Traumatic Stress Disorder in 1980. My investigation had been ongoing for nine years before I came across by chance the book by an ophthalmologist Ross Traquair, whilst browsing in the basement library of the Sydney Eye Hospital.

A recursive investigation, doing the same thing every time to look for the same thing, 'collecting observations, collecting thoughts, learning as you go', can only proceed very slowly — it depends on 'who turns up' as a patient and why. Nothing basically clever, just hum-drum repetition to see if some recognisable consistent pattern would ever emerge.

A consistent abnormal pattern, a new clinical finding, did emerge, very slowly:

'When those people who were reporting abnormal persistent peripheral oscillopsia on visual testing were asked about any fright-

ening experiences in the past, they all were also reporting an abnormal-in-form persistently recurrent, re-experiencing, flashing-back
memory of the experiences during the moment of a sudden traumatic event. And vice versa: those who reported one of the two
abnormal symptoms also reported the other. And this association
of two abnormal symptoms, one of an abnormality of vision and
one of an abnormal form of a recurring flashing back memory of a
frightening event remained invariant, unchanging over time.

When a consistent pattern between two or more seemingly
unrelated abnormal phenomena emerges, one suspects some
abnormal central pattern generator, some continuous mechanism,
responsible for maintaining the consistent pattern.

This abnormal-in-form, persistently recurrent, re-experiencing,
flashing-back memory, when recalled, was a vivid *sensorial and physical re-experiencing, a re-living,* of the frightening experience that
had caused their anxiety disorder—it was not just a *recollection of an
account* of what had happened and how they had felt.

A consistent pattern had emerged of two uniquely abnormal
symptoms being inseparably linked together. Some of the people
with these two inseparably linked abnormal symptoms *did* satisfy
the criteria for PTSD as described in the APA's DSM and WHO's
ICD, and many *did not* satisfy the criteria for PTSD in either: this
consistent pattern of two inseparable symptoms was not, and still is
not, part of the APA's or the WHO's definitions of a PTSD.

But, if a consistent pattern is found, then one is always and
earnestly on the lookout for an exception to prove that it is not a
consistent pattern, perhaps just a series of coincidences looking like
a consistent pattern. One does not want to end up with any flawed
argument, or flawed conclusion. However, one cannot prove anything is a consistent pattern; one can only say that it has passed all
the tests so far to disprove it as a consistent pattern. But in medicine,
'nothing is always, nothing is never'. In Chapter Four, we find that
one exception had turned up — some sixteen thousand miles away,
in Massachusetts, USA — but it is 'an exception' that cannot quite

refute the consistency of 'this pattern' found here. The accumulated evidentiary clinical findings allow one to posit that it most probably is a consistent pattern, a unique-in-form pattern of two linked abnormal symptoms. There were also people with a history of a very frightening event that was followed by a persisting anxiety disorder, but these people were *not reporting persistent peripheral oscillopsia on testing*, regardless of how anxious they were, and they were *not reporting a persistently recurrent abnormal re-experiencing (re-living) flashback memory of the moment of the event that had caused their anxiety disorder*. Many of those people did report intrusive distressing memories of one or more distressing events they had experienced in the past, but the distressing, intrusive memories were not recalled in any abnormal re-experiencing form of memory recall, just as normal-in-form *accounts* of what had happened, terrible events for them as they had been, and not memories of the event(s) they liked or wished to recall.

Some of these people *without the visual and memory abnormalities* also appeared to satisfy the criteria for PTSD as described in the APA's DSM and the WHO's ICD, but not all, i.e. the DSM and ICD definitions of PTSD did not discriminate between the two groups described here—those with and those without the two unique, abnormal symptoms. Some with PTSD of either group who did not qualify for PTSD with DSM or ICD did qualify for one or other of the DSM and ICD 'Trauma- and Stressor-Related Disorders'. Neither DSM nor ICD, in their lists of criteria for PTSD, say anything about a unique form of persistent peripheral oscillopsia and a uniquely abnormal form of recurrent abnormal flashback memory occurring together. So: the DSM and ICD descriptions of PTSD are inconsistent with the fully-testable-by-anyone evidentiary clinical findings coming from this simple clinical investigation – PTSD needed redefining if it were to make any common clinical sense.

But: the DSM and ICD descriptions were never intended to define a specific clinical entity. As we have seen above, they were only intended to define '*who, amongst the many ex-service personnel* *suffering from a persisting anxiety disorder caused by the Vietnam War combat-related mentally traumatic ev*ents' should and should not receive compensation. For those who did warrant compensation, their disorder was to be called PTSD. For those who didn't warrant compensation, their disorder would be called something else. At the time, in 1980, in the aftermath of The Vietnam War, this was a decent, much-needed thing for the APA to do. The APA and WHO descriptions of PTSD were never intended to be fully testable, clinically evidential-based definitions of what an anxiety disorder caused by an experience of a mentally traumatic event actually is. So, if much is to rest on the clinical evidence-based being described here and provide a clinically rigorous definition of 'PTSD', then the evidence-base must be clear and precise. Chapter Three explains in detail 'a unique abnormally formed recurrent re-experiencing flashing-back memory', and Chapter Four explains in detail 'persistent peripheral oscillopsia'. These two invariant and inseparable symptoms obviously are not 'new' symptoms; they must have been around 'forever', but it seems they have not been recognised and characterised in detail, not given an exclusive name before, and not seen to be unique, invariant, and inseparably linked. Their pattern, their linked presence, and details of their unique features, had turned up by chance: serendipitously.

A unique and independent contribution to the nature of persistent peripheral oscillopsia, independently researched and written by the contributing author, Psychologist Professor Brenden Dellar, comes later, following Chapter Four.

CHAPTER THREE

What exactly is a 'persistently recurrent abnormal re-experiencing flashback memory recall'? (And a note on Persistent Complex Bereavement Disorder.)

A preparatory note: At no stage in the diagnosis or treatment of any PTSD is it *necessary* for the person with PTSD to reveal to anyone what had caused their PTSD or reveal the contents of any recurrent abnormal re-experiencing flashback. They may want to reveal it, even talk about it, *but they don't have to if they prefer not to.* What matters in diagnosis and treatment of PTSD is the *form* of the recurrent abnormal re-experiencing flashback—how it comes, when it comes, how it makes one feel when it comes, and, whether there is a positive Visual Test result for persistent peripheral oscillopsia.

A normally formed 'ordinary' everyday memory is: 'being aware of, i.e. 'conscious of, noticing and experiencing something', and contemporaneously, 'laying down a memory engram', meaning an account of what one is conscious of, noticing, and experiencing. A memory engram is a hypothetical permanent change in the brain accounting for the existence of memory, a memory trace. The conscious perception of something and the laying down of the account of it, the memory engram of it, occur contemporaneously. The normally laid-down memory engram may last less than a few seconds or may last up to a lifetime. When the memory is recalled normally, it is recalled as *an account* of what was being aware of, an account of having been conscious of the something, having noticed, experienced the something. Giving an account of the something is not giving a re-experiencing of the something, and it is not a re-living of the something.

A recurrent abnormal re-experiencing flashback memory recall is an abnormally formed memory engram being recalled. An abnormally formed engram gives a memory recall in which there is an abnormal re-experiencing of, not just an account of, the experiences during a particular circumscribed moment of the past, a moment when the person was experiencing an unexpected sudden surge of high anxiety, 'a mental shock'. The memory engram of the happenings of that circumscribed moment could not be processed normally for a reason we come to later, hence it had to be stored as an improperly processed memory engram of the experiences of that circumscribed moment, and, whenever it is recalled, it can only be recalled as an improperly processed memory engram of that moment: recalled as an abnormal emotional, physical and sensorial re-experiencing 'flashback' memory of PTSD type 1. (See later for the necessary subdivision of 'PTSD' into PTSD type 1 and PTSD type 2).

The recall of the improperly processed engram of that moment is always in the unique, abnormal form of not only remembering but also of an actual re-experiencing, an actual re-living of the sights that were seen (noticed), of the thoughts that were thought (noticed), of the emotions of fear and anxiety and disgust that were felt (noticed), a re-living of the physical sensations of what was happening bodily (noticed), a re-living of the physical sensations of pain (noticed), a re-hearing of the physical sensations of sounds (noticed), and a re-smelling of the smell (noticed)—in other words, a re-living of all the sensations of what had been consciously noticed and experienced of what was noticed only during that moment of the sudden surge of high anxiety, the mental shock. In other words, not everything that happened during that circumscribed moment may have been noticed; hence, not everything that happened was remembered.

That momentary sudden surge of high anxiety, the 'mental shock' damaged the brain; it did something physical—it changed the way a part of the brain functioned, from a normal way of functioning to an abnormal way of functioning—giving rise to a brain with an anxiety disorder of PTSD type 1: i.e. a brain with (i), an abnormally formed engram of the experiences noticed during that circumscribed moment of a surge of high anxiety, an abnormally-formed engram that is repeatedly re-called as an abnormally-formed 're-experiencing engram, (ii), a persistently high level of anxiety, and (iii), persistent peripheral oscillopsia, present whenever tested for.

Inserted here, for the sake of the clarity of the story, we 'jump the gun' for a moment:

Later, in Chapters Eight and Nine, we come to some of the inferences that can be drawn from evidentiary clinical findings. They include, (i), of how the brain was 'damaged' by an epigenetic insertion on the right side, not the left side, giving rise to PTSD type 1 (not PTSD type 2), (ii), of how some, not all people with PTSD type 1, can be totally cured by EMDR treatment that reverses the epigenetic insertion; and why some people with PTSD type 1 cannot be cured at all by EMDR treatment; and, (iii), of how some people are more likely than other people to get PTSD type 1 when they experience a mental shock.

Recurrent abnormal flashbacks of PTSD type 1 (we are still coming to a PTSD type 1 and a PTSD type 2) are a uniquely abnormal mental phenomenon; they recur only when wide awake. They are not bad dreams, they are not nightmares, and they are not dissociation phenomena. In response to focussing attention on the re-experiencing features of the recurrent abnormal flashback, there may be some transient preoccupation, hampering awareness of the surrounding social environment for the duration of the abnormal flashback, mimicking 'dissociation'. Unique features and examples of recurrent abnormal flashbacks are described in detail later in this chapter.

"Dissociation phenomena" are defined as 'disruptions of consciousness (that is, disruptions of full awareness), of identity, or of memory, or of physical actions, or of the environment—any one or more of these. They are not a frequent feature of people with PTSD type 1. They are called derealisation and or depersonalization phenomena. If a person experiences many dissociation symptoms, they may be diagnosed with a Dissociative Disorder. Forms of transient dissociation are associated with anxiety. They can occur in response to a 'mental shock', so a sudden surge of intense anxiety, a 'mental shock with transient dissociation' may engender a PTSD type 1 and or a PTSD type 2 (details later) and a transient dissociation may also occur at some stage in someone with a PTSD type 1 and or a PTSD type 2. There is a rare form of Permanent Dissociative Disorder with persisting distressingly altered awareness. It is suspected of being associated with some form of temporary or permanent physical brain dysfunction of some unknown physical cause and nature (cf. the visual phenomena of migraines). It has no abnormal flashbacks and no oscillopsia associated with it. It is suspected of being a rare form of transient or permanent post-traumatic stress disorder, but with no clinical evidence that it is related in form to what is discussed here as post-traumatic stress disorder. So, a recurrent abnormal flashback is NOT a dissociation phenomenon: it has its own unique defining characteristics.

Many people speak of having experienced a mental shock. Not all who experience a mental shock develop an anxiety disorder or develop a persistently recurrent abnormal re-experiencing flashback memory of the experience of the event that triggered the mental shock. Not everyone experiences a mental shock in response to a sudden realization of being in imminent danger or in response to experiencing intense disgust, or in response to experiencing intense emotional distress, whether experiencing an intensely mentally traumatic event or not. Not everyone takes the trouble to discover the reason for their having had a panic attack.

Some details of a persistently recurrent abnormal re-experiencing flashback memory recall, an abnormal re-experiencing (an experiential) flashback of an abnormally formed memory engram.

Anyone with the form of PTSD type 1, i.e. who does have persistently recurrent abnormally formed re-experiencing flashback memory recalls, knows perfectly well what their own flashback is and how it makes them feel. Many people have given details of the form and the content of their own one, or of more than one, of their own abnormal re-experiencing flashback memories. Not all people are willing to talk about them, and for many good reasons: talking about them means re-evoking and re-experiencing them, bringing back the sudden distressing anxiety: perhaps a surge of anger, a surge of shame or revulsion, a return of a frightening scene, a return of physical pain, or a distressing noise, or a distressing smell—some or all of these.

At the other extreme of the spectrum of severity of PTSD type 1, some people *do not appear to know* that they have a persistently recurrent abnormal re-experiencing flashback of PTSD type 1 or *do not recognise it as abnormal until asked about the detail of its form.* People may not know they have any form of PTSD type 1 or PTSD type 2 either, until asked about the level of their everyday anxiety and having or not having persistent peripheral oscillopsia on testing. There certainly can be, has to be, a clinically insignificant PTSD type 1 and or clinically insignificant PTSD type 2.

This wide range of the severity of abnormal flashbacks—a spectrum of severity ranging from there being very many abnormal flashbacks and all of distressing and disabling severity, to there being just one that is merely trivially upsetting—goes hand in hand with the wide spectrum of the severity and life-long disruptiveness of an anxiety disorder PTSD type 1 itself. This is an issue somewhat interfering with intuition: some PTSDs are terribly severe at one end of the spectrum of severity, and some PTSDs are hardly noticeable at the lowest end of the spectrum of severity—such a wide spectrum of severity of PTSD tends to 'debase the currency' of severe PTSD for those with the most severe forms of PTSD. DSM and ICD try to maintain a high face value of PTSD currency for the very good reasons they had been faced with at the time—they needed a disorder that was defined as being of sufficient severity to warrant lifetime compensation. The spectrum of severity of post-traumatic stress disorder appears to be one of Nature's many continuums, where adjacent elements are not perceptibly different from each other, but the extremes are distinct. It is not biologically plausible or clinically practical to artificially divide one of Nature's continuums and place a quantifiable line between the severe having one name and the not severe having another name, as is tried in DSM and ICD.

The experiences that were remembered during that circumscribed moment of mental shock are not remembered normally nor recalled normally (unless and until the PTSD type 1 is permanently and completely curd with successful EMDR—see just below). The abnormal memory engram of the experiences during that moment of mental shock had been abnormally laid down, the abnormally formed engram having been abnormally processed during that moment of the surge of high anxiety. For some people, but not all people, and dependent on their genetic make-up (their genotype), the abnormally formed engram of the noticed happenings during that momentary period of time can be correctly processed and then recalled normally by properly performed EMDR treatment. We define 'properly performed 'EMDR treatment' in Chapter Eleven. We come to what constitutes a permanent cure or a permanent failure to cure PTSD type 1 later in Chapter Eleven.

What follows here are some given accounts of what has been 'physically and mentally' re-experienced during a persistently recurrent abnormal re-experiencing flashback of an abnormally-formed memory engram.

The re-experienced **anxiety** during that moment: the awareness of the *physical* shaking, shivering, thumping heartbeat, sweating, the emotion of fear, panic, disgust; and re-experienced **thoughts** of 'those people have been killed', 'I'm going to die', 'I'll never get out of this', she's going to kill me', 'he's going to rape me', 'I couldn't believe all this would ever happen'…

The experienced **re-seeing** aspects of what was being seen (visually noticed) during that moment: an eidetic picture, meaning mental images having unusual vividness and detail, as if still actually visible, a vivid mental picture seen, "… out there just where it was in the visual field at the time …" The eidetic picture may be a detailed still-picture in full colour, or a constantly re-running brief video-clip in full colour, of all or of just some aspects of what had been seen (noticed) during the moment of the mental shock, during the surge of anxiety. If the event occurred in the dark, then the scene will be one of darkness. Some examples are: 'a threatening gun being menacingly pointed; a grinning aggressive face of an angry superior at work while being reprimanded; a bloodied corpse and body parts at an accident site, at a bomb site, at a murder site or in a burnt-out building; the background region of the room, with blowing curtains; near total darkness as it was at the time; something that was incidentally being noticed while listening to an intensely frightening phone call; the face of a mother seen by a child, who is in the middle of a panic attack as mother is coming to give comfort; a vehicle seen approaching immediately prior to an unavoidable collision; a shattered windscreen seen immediately after a collision; the face of a loved one in their coffin; the face of a loved one in agonising pain; the rapidly approaching engulfing flames in woodland or in a house; the office surround of where one had been working and noticed in detail while having a sudden heart attack; a battlefield colleague who was standing next to one a second ago but now writhing and bleeding to death on the ground; a child, or a comrade being blown up by a bomb or a landmine; the colour of the walls of the room in which one was being raped.'

The physical **re-hearing** of aspects of the awareness of what was heard during that moment. Some examples are: the distinct words being spoken; the screams; the screech of brakes; the crumbling metal; the gunfire; the breathing and grunts of a rapist; the crunch of collapsing buildings during an earthquake; the screech of a hurricane as it lifts the roof; the gasps and groans of a dying injured child or comrade...

The physical **re-feeling** aspects of what had been noticed as physically felt during that moment. Examples are: 'the pain; the penetration; the choking; the falling; the physical torturing; the tears, the screams...

The physical **re-smelling, and re-tasting** aspects of what was noticed to have been smelled or tasted during that moment. Examples are: 'the petrol; the putrefaction; the faeces; the smoke...'. (Recurrent smells and tastes are common and somewhat less specific.)

A 'special case': **Persistent Complex Bereavement Disorder**. A recurrent abnormal flashback of a frightening eidetic image of a loved one, at or near the time of their death, the sight having been engendered by a mental shock at that moment. And perhaps in addition, at different times, brief and quite normal-looking (veridical, truthful) 'hallucinations', 'apparitions', quite unrelated to the PTSD type 1, of 'seeing the loved one in the house or garden or elsewhere as they were when alive and well'. These people will have persistent anxiety and persistent peripheral oscillopsia and will require a trial of EMDR to help them get rid of their PTSD type 1 as an essential part of helping them through their grief.

It may not be easy, but the abnormal flashback must be distinguished from recurrent *normally formed* intrusive, distressing memories of traumatic events. They must also be distinguished from distressing dreams and nightmares of traumatic events. They must be distinguished from veridical (truthful) hallucinations of seeing recently deceased loved ones as they were in life. Many normally formed intrusive distressing memories of traumatic events may be intermingled at any time with abnormally formed abnormal re-experiencing flashbacks. There are several other features of persistently recurrent and abnormal re-experiencing flashbacks: every abnormally formed flashback is unique to anyone that any one person has had.

There can be several different abnormal flashbacks, occurring together or separately, of various memories from different moments of distinct mental shocks. These can arise from the experience of just one traumatic event or from multiple experiences from one or many traumatic events. The separate traumatic events may have been separated in time by seconds, minutes, days, or decades. Each separate abnormal-in-form re-experiencing flashback represents a separate module of PTSD type 1. Each separate normal-in-form intensely distressing flashback represents a separate module of PTSD type 2.

The frequency of the recurrence of the abnormal-in-form re-experiencing flashbacks can vary from many times a day to once or twice a year. Each one can last from a few seconds to several minutes. They tend to lessen in frequency over time but are unlikely to lessen significantly in intensity (unless treated with exposure therapy—see later). When left untreated or are untreatable, then attempts are usually made to get rid of them by mental distraction, perhaps aided by some physical action, such as mouthing an expletive, hitting a wall with a fist, smashing a glass, self-harming with a cigarette burn to the arm; taking a swift-acting drug or swig of a strong alcohol drink...

Children of five or six and over can experience and clearly describe recurrent abnormal flashbacks, as they can clearly describe persistent peripheral oscillopsia during The Visual Test.

All the contents of any one abnormally formed re-experiencing flashback are remembered in normal form following successful EMDR treatment for that specific memory. The abnormally formed engram, when processed to normal engram form by successful EMDR treatment, may remain recurrently intrusive, despite being in normal form, and very distressing because of the content of the factual, existential experience.

The Visual Test for persistent peripheral oscillopsia is specific, reliable, and sensitive to detect the presence or absence of an abnormal flashback of PTSD type 1, or of any remaining fragment of one, at any time, and regardless of the time since the abnormally formed memory was last evoked.

CHAPTER FOUR

What, exactly, is the uniquely abnormal visual phenomenon, 'persistent peripheral oscillopsia'?

It is *a clear clinical signal, regardless of clinical noise, for the presence or absence of PTSD type 1.* (We come to PTSD type 1 later in Chapter 5)

Persistent peripheral oscillopsia is an illusory visual perception of persistent rhythmical movement of stationary objects seen (usually only) in the *periphery* of the visual field while maintaining a steady gaze at a stationary object straight ahead, i.e. seeing persistent rhythmical movement that is not real, not present. This abnormal visual phenomenon was called 'a stammering of perception in the periphery of the visual field' when it was first described (as far as we know) and written in a book, by an ophthalmologist in 1946. The ophthalmologist was reporting in his book what some ex-soldiers with Traumatic Neurosis had told him they observed themselves. The ex-soldiers with Traumatic Neurosis had all reported this same thing to the ophthalmologist as the ophthalmologist was conducting routine visual fields tests of the ex-soldiers' visual fields.

A simple Visual Test has been devised to detect the presence or absence of *persistent peripheral oscillopsia* in anyone over the age of five or six years. The simple test is sensitive, reliable, and specific for PTSD type 1. (We come to PTSD type 1 in Chapter 5) The simple test can be performed by anyone on anyone who is not blind or uncooperative. It is briefly described here.

The simple Visual Test for the presence or absence of persistent peripheral oscillopsia. More details are given in Chapter Ten.

The person being tested is seated. The examiner stands a meter or so directly in front of them. The person being examined covers their left eye, and with the right eye, they steadily fixate their gaze on the left eye of the examiner, who has his right eye covered. The person is asked to fixate their gaze on the left eye of the examiner for ten seconds, and, at the same time, take notice of what appears to start happening, immediately or within a few seconds, to the stationary extended left arm of the examiner.

'Steadily fixating' means keeping their left eye covered and keeping their right eye firmly fixed on the open left eye of the examiner for ten seconds, without blinking or glancing elsewhere, even momentarily. The examiner monitors the person's steady gaze throughout the ten seconds, with his open left eye fixed on the open right eye of the person being examined.

At the end of the ten seconds, the examiner lowers his left arm and asks the person to demonstrate with their right arm how the examiner's left arm appeared to them during the ten seconds of their steady gaze.

How the examiner appears through the right eye of the person being tested.

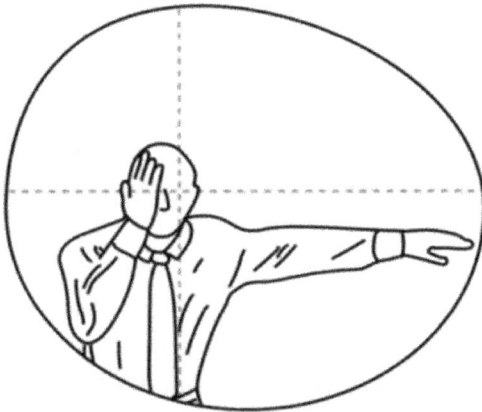

Picture by Silas Tym

For some people with peripheral oscillopsia, there appear to be up-and-down or similar oscillations of some aspect of the examiner's left arm from the outset of the test, i.e. up-and-down oscillations of the whole arm, or just peripherally from the forearm, or just from the hand, or only just the fingers. For some people, this appearance of oscillation can start as soon as their steady eye-fixation starts; for others, the oscillations always appear only after a few seconds of steady eye-fixation, i.e. there is a constant delay in onset which, for each person, is always the same delay on subsequent Visual Tests. This *delay in the onset of oscillations* can vary from one second to six or seven seconds from the start of steady fixation. (The illusory perception of the oscillations will persist for as long as steady fixation is maintained on the examiner's stationary left eye by the person being tested, if the examiner were to keep his left arm stationary and extended, and his left eye fixated on the person's right eye, for more than the ten seconds.)

For any one person, the **oscillations** at each Visual Test have a constant *frequency*, usually of approximately two to three waves or cycles per second. For any one person, the oscillations, at each

Visual Test, have a constant *amplitude*, usually of a few degrees or possibly up to 45 or more degrees. For any one person, the oscillations, at each Visual Test, have a constant *range over the visual field,* i.e. it might be limited to the tips of the examiner's fingers (the very periphery of the visual field) or extend to his whole arm (i.e. more extensively, virtually throughout the whole visual field). (More details of the simple test are given in Chapter Ten.)

This visual test was the final form of visual testing, not the first form of visual testing, devised in the thirty-year exploratory clinical investigation into any abnormality of vision following trauma.

(See four paragraphs below: the independent investigation into the clinical evidence for persistent oscillopsia conducted by Assistant Professor of Psychology, Dr Brendon Dellar, for his PhD thesis in 2006.)

Persistent peripheral oscillopsia is not found in any other disorder, mental or physical—but with the usual caveat: 'nothing is never, nothing is always in any branch of medicine'.

*There is one case report by a Dr Jacome, a neurologist in Turners Falls, Massachusetts. He reported:

Migrainous Binocular Peripheral Oscillopsia. (Neurology' 2013; 4(2)). Viz. An 18-year-old woman with intermittent attacks of migraine and a recent onset of bilateral persistent peripheral oscillopsia when visually fixating on stationary objects. The young woman's oscillopsia settled within a few weeks in response to antimigraine medication.

I spoke by phone with Dr Jacome. Dr Jacome said there was no evidence of PTSD of any sort in the young woman, nor any other eye, ear or nervous system abnormality detected other than recurrent migraine. Dr Jacome had treasured his one exception and published his one-and-only case because he could find no similar case report anywhere in the literature. He allowed me to mention his case in this book. Migraine is notorious for temporarily, sometimes not so temporarily, and sometimes permanently disrupting virtually any aspect of neurological functioning, especially vision. I have not seen any similar case report.

Unknown to me at the time, in 2001, the nature and correlates of persistent peripheral oscillopsia had been independently investigated at length by Assistant Professor of Psychology, Dr Brendon Dellar, for his PhD Thesis, published in 2006. Professor Dellar introduces an abstract of his thesis.

Adjunct Professor of Psychology, Brendon Dellar, Ph D, Presently Director, Cygnet Clinic, Perth, and Adjunct Professor, Curtin University, Perth. Western Australia.

Abstract of the PhD thesis of Brendon Joseph Dellar, Curtin University, Perth, Western Australia, published in 2006. (272 pages. 2 files. 16739 Dellar 20B 202006 20. espace.curtin.edu.au)

This thesis was concerned with investigating a visual-illusionary phenomenon that co-occurs with post-traumatic anxiety symptoms. More specifically, individuals who report recurring specific memories of a fearful event (RSM) also tend to report a persistent illusion of movement (PIM) upon prolonged visual fixation.

The development of a visual test (i-Test) designed to reliably elicit PIM has enabled research to be conducted on the nature and correlates of this type of visual disturbance. The present research aimed:

i) To develop a standard protocol for assessment of PIM and RSM.

ii) To test the reliability of the i-Test in eliciting PIM in a student sample.

iii) To test the predictive relationship between dissociation and anxiety symptoms with PIM and RSM.

iv) To formulate and test a hypothesis regarding a mechanism underlying PIM. The first study screened 142 participants for RSM and PIM using self-administered questionnaires.

Summary by a/prof Dellar of his 2006 thesis:

Psychological Investigations into Persistent Peripheral Oscillopsia in Traumatic Stress

In 2001, I stumbled across an interesting research article when studying as a postgraduate student at Curtin University, Perth. This article was authored by Dr Robert Tym, Consultant Psychiatrist,

(Tym, R, Dyke, M, & McGrath, G. (2000) Journal of Anxiety Disorders 14(4) 377-395.)

The fascinating part of this research was that it was on a novel symptom in posttraumatic stress conditions that had been mentioned sporadically through various citations during the last century. All of these were observations of people returning from war or recent witnessing of traumatic events that cited visual problems. The problems were with wavy, stammering, or pulsating vision, known by the medical profession as oscillopsia. Most of the documented literature was on observation of this reported symptom, but apart from descriptions, there were no in-depth scientific investigations into what causes unstable vision in traumatised individuals. Most of what was understood about oscillopsia came from ophthalmological research. In this area of inquiry, oscillopsia is linked to uncontrollable eye movements medically referred to as nystagmus. This condition is usually the result of some form of neurobiological problems observed from birth or through some other form of acquired injury (whether it be disease or acquired brain injuries). What was known was that if you were born with Nystagmus, you were less likely to have unstable vision, predominantly linked to the ability of a developing brain to adjust and compensate for the side-to-side swinging motion of the eyes. The group of people who acquired nystagmus was almost always presented with oscillopsia. Looking back at Dr Tym's observations, the traumatic patients he was documenting were also presenting with acquired oscillopsia through the experience of trauma, resulting in intrusive memories and persistent anxiety linked to the event. My interest in this area was in the parallels between what was emerging as an effective treatment for Post-Traumatic Stress Disorder (PTSD) using Eye-Movement Desensitisation and Reprocessing (EMDR) and the treatment of the well-understood ophthalmological condition of nystagmus with oscillopsia. While at this time, EMDR had controversial debates over how and why this technique worked, the condition of acquired nystagmus was being treated by Orthoptists with eye exercises that remarkably resemble EMDR. This was the moment when I realised that oscillopsia cited by Dr Tym was linked to EMDR as a successful trauma treatment while for many years, a separate branch of medicine had been treating nystagmus-based oscillopsia by similar methods. The research at this stage was a single study published in the Journal of Anxiety Disorders by Tym, Dyck & McGrath (2001). The remarkable finding in this study was that while oscillopsia appeared to present in people with other disorders (specifically panic disorder), every single person with a formal diagnosis of PTSD had tested positive for persistent peripheral oscillopsia. No other diagnosed condition had specifically presented with this visual disturbance.

All this documented evidence was compelling enough to com-
mence a series of experiments in a visual perceptual laboratory
I had set up at university. The aim was to understand the mechanisms that might explain rather than just describe this form
of oscillopsia. The idea of visual symptoms to diagnose mental
health conditions was sceptically received by academic scholars
at the time, mostly because of polarisation of views on EMDR
and the fact that visual symptoms in psychiatric diagnosis were
firmly conceived as a psychodynamic projective test (e.g., Ror-
schach famous ink blot tests). From a scientific point of view,
new symptoms are often explained by phenomena that have
already been discovered. Unsurprisingly, in this case, the investigations followed the same orthodox view that this form of visual
instability is probably the result of eye movements (at one level
or another) or the stimulus used in the testing.

Explanation 1: Oscillopsia as an established nystagmus symptom.

The first explanation was one mentioned earlier in the discussion
of known ophthalmological causes of oscillopsia. The explanation
that there is a link between acquired brain injury from trauma
resulting in a traumatic symptom is easy to understand. Nystagmus occurs largely in two groups of people, the latter group being
the one most likely to experience oscillopsia. The first group is
those with congenital (i.e. From birth) nystagmus, and they
tend to adjust and stabilise their vision through neurobiological development that accommodates and essentially cancels out
any perception of movement that would ordinarily plague those
with uncontrollable eye movements. The group with acquired
brain injury at a later stage tends to have difficulties with oscillopsia. On the surface, this is an appealing first explanation for

why there appeared to be a strong link between traumatic stress conditions and oscillopsia, given that a proportion of people involved in accident-related trauma may acquire a brain injury and by natural extension of this, they would be more likely to have oscillopsia as a result. The other exaptational (the process by which features acquire functions for which they were not originally adapted or selected) was that exposure to drugs and alcohol to regulate emotions in people with PTSD might be a second reason why oscillopsia is associated with traumatic anxiety. This had been investigated, and although there were observations of subjects spontaneously displaying nystagmus-like movements, none of them had histories of drug or alcohol abuse, nor did their traumatic incidence involve a motor-vehicle or some other form of head injury that would explain the onset of stammering vision. Furthermore, most of the subjects with PTSD had clear oscillopsia but demonstrated no nystagmus. Ophthalmological research being carried out independently by Dr Tym and his colleagues in ophthalmology also confirmed this. The stammering vision is not the cause of acquired nystagmus.

Explanation 2: Oscillopsia is a form of Autokinetic Phenomenon.

An interesting explanation for PTSD oscillopsia was related to the experimental design used in the original 2001 published article. The stimulus used to induce oscillopsia was created by Dr Tym and consisted of a black-uniformed background with a light-yellow strip in the centre that stood vertically upward, resembling the letter "i" later named the iTest for this reason. The dot point on the central strip was where the subjects were asked to fix their gaze and those with traumatic oscillopsia tended to see the bottom strip of the rectangle wave from side to side. During testing, the stimulus was placed in a head stabilisation frame at a standard distance to minimise the effect of head movement or unintentional movement of handheld iTest by the examiner.

(A test no longer used.)

The interesting history of illusionary movement was in the context of the Autokinetic Movement Phenomenon (AMP). This illusion induced by fixation on a central high-contract stimulus on a uniform black background. In most cases, laboratories investigating this AK Movement are in dark rooms where a single point of light is observed, and the subject is asked to fixate on it. Usually, the light remains stationary for a few seconds upon steady gaze, and then appears to move about. The illusionary movement can be pronounced in some people and does not have any relationship to the organic nystagmus described above. The AMP illusion is well documented and has been linked to our visual system's need for a context to establish visual stability (e.g., you need some form of visual landscape or at least more than one point of reference). This illusion has been used to explain some Unidentified Flying Objects (UFOs) where the dark sky has one point of reference, such as the moon without enough star light to produce a point of reference. This appeared very similar to the iTest originally used to induce oscillopsia. Nearly 80 years ago, it was studied as a method for psychiatric diagnosis, but since then, did not receive much attention. Dr Tym's subsequent studies of Traumatic Oscillopsia have used stimuli with various contexts without the uniform black background used in the original research. The use of an extended arm as a stimulus-inducing oscillopsia, as documented by Dr Tym, is not consistent with the necessary environment to induce illusionary movement in AMP.

Explanation 3 – Oscillopsia as a symptom of Pulse

The initial research on oscillopsia in the 2001 published article stated that the rate of oscillopsia was approximately 1 to 3Hz and that any movement faster than this would not be clinically relevant. The other unanticipated finding of the 2001 study was that people with panic disorder also reported persistent illusionary movement at this rate. Aside from both being anxiety disorders, there is much in common between these two diagnoses and high levels of co-morbidity, making it difficult to separate. The pulsatile hypothesis was based on the observed rate of the illusionary movement (1 to 3Hz). This corresponds to a heart rate range of 60bpm to 180bpm and is well understood to be a symptom that creates disturbances for people with anxious arousal symptoms in panic disorder and PTSD. There have been other established rhymical perceptual symptoms caused by sensitivity to cardiovascular symptoms, most notably in Pulsatile Tinnitus, where the individual with anxious arousal hears the persistent thumping of their heart. If this was the cause of the Oscillopsia, then manipulation of heart rate through exertion would change the rate of Oscillopsia accordingly. The problem we faced was that the documented 1 to 3Hz was an estimation that the subjects in previous studies gave when asked by the examiner how fast the rhythm of the oscillopsia was. To overcome this, we created a randomised metronome that produced rhymical sounds and a random point between 0.2Hz and 10Hz with a dial that could change the tempo of the metronome in steps of 0.2Hz (not exceeding 10Hz or less than 0.2Hz). The subjects were asked to adjust the metronome only if they reported rhymical movement consistent with the oscillopsia symptom. All subjects were required to increase their pulse rate by exercising on a bicycle to 80% of the maximum cardiovascular load for their age and gender. Once the pulse rate was sufficiently increased, the subject was asked to repeat the visual test for oscillopsia. Half the group did this in reverse order to cancel out some experimental errors that can occur from doing a certain task before another. The results were not expected. Not only did the increase in pulse rate have no corresponding increase in oscillopsia rate, but the effect was that exercise prolonged the time it took for the oscillopsia to reappear. At resting rate, individuals perceiving movement usually do so in a few seconds (around 3 seconds on average). Having increased their pulse rate added 10 seconds or more to the onset of the illusionary movement. It appeared that the oscillopsia was initiated once the subjects returned to a resting level heart rate (irrespective of their own resting level heart rate). The other important finding was that the rate of oscillopsia through the randomised metronome was remarkably consistent, with all subjects reporting around 1Hz. This was far more uniform than expected and demonstrated the consistency of the observed oscillopsia symptoms between individuals, making them easier to test for.

Explanation 4: Oscillopsia is a cortical symptom of traumatic anxiety.

This last explanation is the one that fits best. Previously, we have looked for observable peripheral symptoms such as eye movements or increased pulse rate to explain this symptom. The largest correlation is between those reporting traumatic re-experiencing symptoms (i.e. intrusive visual memories or flashbacks) with persistent oscillopsia. There has been a method of testing for cortical arousal through the perception of flicker in intermittent lights. Research in anxiety conditions had already established the link between high cortical arousal and a lower threshold for detecting flicker in non-incandescent lighting. Some researchers even went as far as to propose that Agoraphobia in Panic Disorder may be at least exacerbated by an anxious person's sensitivity to flicker in fluorescent lighting found in many shopping malls and supermarkets. Using a Critical Flicker Frequency device, we were able to establish that the intrusive traumatic and recurring memories in those with traumatic stress disorders did demonstrate both oscillopsia and an increased sensitivity to flicker. This flicker sensitivity is related to activity in the visual cortex and related cortical systems, pointing toward a unified theory that oscillopsia is related to traumatic changes in brain activity rather than a well-established visual illusion or ophthalmological mechanism. This form of oscillopsia is novel and related to a range of symptoms that are unique to what is now shown by Dr Robert Tym to be PTSD type 1 as described by him.

CHAPTER FIVE

FORMAL DEFINITIONS of PTSD type 1 and PTSD type 2.

A clinical observational consequence: there must be two different forms of the 'anxiety disorder PTSD', not just one: the two disorders are superficially clinically very similar but neurologically, genomically, and biologically very different.

A new but simple taxonomy (classification) of an anxiety disorder PTSD type 1 and an anxiety disorder PTSD type 2.

The anxiety disorder **PTSD type 1,** a categorical disorder, always has two unique clinical features, and it cannot resolve spontaneously over time—if it cannot respond to treatment, it persists for the rest of life. The anxiety disorder **PTSD type 2,** a dimensional disorder, has no unique clinical features; it can respond to treatment, and can resolve spontaneously over time, but not always does, depending on mentally traumatic circumstances that prolong its presence.

Respect is paid here to the many experienced psychiatrists and psychologists who have contributed their own taxonomy, their own branded types, and subtypes of post-traumatic stress disorders, including the branded PTSDs of DSM 5 and ICD 11. These other brands are described elsewhere. There are, however, no evidentiary clinical findings cited to suggest those other brands are distinct clinical entities, as are PTSD type 1 and PTSD type 2.

To have arrived where we are today is thanks to the Sixteenth century Dr Thomas Sydenham, The Father of Observational Medicine. He reminded us that: "Nothing in medicine is too insignificant as to not merit attention"; and "It is at the bedside, that is where you learn about disease, put those tomes away". The hitherto all but ignored clinical symptom of persistent peripheral oscillopsia has now been given attention. Many people have been listened to (virtually) "at the bedside" and clinically examined. In this context, the tomes of DSM and ICD have been put away. And thanks, too, to the early 1900's Dr William Osler, The Father of Modern Medicine: he told us: "Just listen to the patients, they are telling you the diagnosis", (assuming one asks the right questions).

William Ockham, the Thirteenth century philosopher, has also been listened to: his immortal 'Occam's Razor' still says, "Plurality must never be posited without necessity; the simplest solution tends to be the right one". But this plurality of two disorders, a PTSD type 1 and a PTSD type 2, is posited with necessity: the evidentiary clinical findings tell us that it is necessarily more complex to have the new taxonomy, a PTSD type 1 and a PTSD type 2, but it does succinctly comply with the evidentiary clinical findings. So, this bifaceted indexing of two PTSDs rather than one, does, as it must, comply with the immortal Occam's Razor.

William of Ockham was a Franciscan Friar and philosopher. His name immortalised the small English village of Ockham, Surrey, UK, where most people say he was born in 1285; others say he was a Yorkshireman, born in Ockham, Yorkshire, in 1285. His clear thinking is certainly more like that of a Yorkshireman than of someone from Surrey. He died in Munich in 1347. His razor is the *lex parsimoniae*, Latin for 'law of parsimony'—'explanations require only what is necessary in light of the evidence'. His razor shaves off all superfluous inferences and explanations, leaving the bare minimum, only the fewest, most plausible and reasonable inferences taken from the evidentiary clinical findings, in this case of two different "PTSDs".

Bearing in mind the human brain and human genomics are complicated, some inferences are drawn from the readily confirmable evidentiary clinical findings given in Chapters Eight and Nine. Perhaps Ockham's razor will allow the inferences given in Chapters Eight and Nine to survive intact, at least for the foreseeable future. Hopefully, there are no superfluous inferences in Chapters Eight and Nine regarding the different biological natures of the two superficially similar but distinctly different PTSD type 1 and PTSD type 2.

PTSD type 1 is a 'categorical disorder' (i.e. 'a disorder that is unique in form), with a wide spectrum of severity varying from person to person. Its diagnosis depends on the invariant (i.e. unchanging) presence of two unique clinical symptoms that are unique to PTSD type 1. Neither symptom appears in any other mental or physical disorder, e.g., not in PTSD type 2. One symptom is of an 'abnormal form of memory recall of a mentally traumatic event', described above, and one symptom is of 'persistent peripheral oscillopsia', described above. The person with PTSD type 1 also has persisting distress and anxiety immediately following a damaging-to-them mental shock, meaning a sudden surge of intense anxiety from sudden fear or sudden disgust from experiencing a mentally traumatic event. The nature of the mentally traumatic event is immaterial. For that person, the experience was sufficient for them to develop a damaging mental shock, and the mental shock, the sudden surge of anxiety, was sufficient to produce their PTSD type 1. The PTSD type 1 is present from the first moment of the mental shock that caused it and cannot resolve spontaneously, i.e. it persists for the remainder of life, regardless of age of onset, unless it can be successfully treated.

After the onset of PTSD type 1 there is always one uniquely abnormal-in-form recurrent recall, an experiential (i.e. re-experiencing, re-living) flashing back memory engram of aspects of the causal event. The abnormally formed memory engram is stored, and it is recurrently recalled in the abnormal form of a flashing back experiential memory engram of the emotional, physical, and sensorial sensations and the memory of aspects of objective happenings that were experienced during the circumscribed moment of the mental shock, i.e. this is the 'abnormal re-experiencing flashback' unique to PTSD type 1.

From the moment of the causal mental shock, there is always the uniquely abnormal visual perceptual phenomenon of persistent peripheral oscillopsia, apparent whenever tested for via the Visual Test (unless the person is blind or uncooperative).

Virtually always, there is also a noticeable persisting level of anxiety that is higher in intensity than is normal for that person. There is always at least one or more persisting non-specific anxiety-related symptoms. These may include, but not necessarily will include, nightmares, hyper-vigilance, exaggerated startle responses, avoidance of external reminders, avoidance of thoughts and feelings associated with the traumatic event, headaches, inattentiveness, insomnia, emotional withdrawal, depressed mood, episodic dissociation, episodic derealization, panic attacks.

PTSD type 1 has not been diagnosed before the age of five years in this clinical investigation (perhaps explained by the concept of 'infantile amnesia').

In those above the age of five or six years with PTSD type 1, the presence or absence of PTSD type 1 can be diagnosed via the simple Visual Test for the presence or absence of persistent peripheral oscillopsia. The test can be performed by anyone, on anyone aged over 5 years or so, who is not blind, and is cooperative.

PTSD type 1 does not resolve spontaneously. If not cured by EMDR treatment (see later), it persists for the rest of life. Its severity in terms of anxiety can be greatly ameliorated by Exposure Therapy, with or without adjuvant anti-anxiety substances.

PTSD type 1 can be present together with other mental disorders, including psychotic disorders, and PTSD type 2 (below), as well as with physical disorders, including traumatic brain injury (TBI).

From person to person, PTSD type 1 can be of any severity, a spectrum of severity ranging from being persistently horrendous, to being 'clinically insignificant': present but virtually unnoticed until attention is drawn to it.

To be precise and reductionist, the anxiety disorder PTSD type 1 is, in essence, the presence of a 'symptom module', 'a unique double symptom', i.e. the presence of a recurrent unique, abnormal re-experiencing form of one circumscribed memory engram, insep-arably linked with, a unique, abnormal form of vision, persistent peripheral oscillopsia. Hence, PTSD type 1 can be mono-modular or multi-modular: i.e. there may be two or more modules of PTSD type 1, each having been caused by different momentary experi-ences of damaging mental shock at different times.

Successful EMDR treatment only removes one module of PTSD type 1 at a time. PTSD type 1 remains present until the last fragment of the last module of PTSD type 1 has been successfully removed by EMDR treatment. Only then is there not the slightest persistent peripheral oscillopsia on testing. Not every person with PTSD type 1 can be helped by EMDR.

With each module of PTSD type 1, there is virtually always a noticeable persisting anxiety of intensity higher than is normal for that person and one or more persisting non-specific anxiety-related symptoms. When the last PTSD type 1 module has been removed, there is no anxiety remaining that is directly attributable to PTSD type 1.

Properly performed EMDR treatment can completely cure *some* people with PTSD type 1 but *not a*ll people with PTSD type 1, and the evidentiary clinical findings are that this success or failure depends on the genotype of the person with the PTSD type 1, i.e. the person with the PTSD type 1 having one of the 'right' genomes, one of the 'right' gen otypes, that can 'allow' EMDR treatment to be effective. EMDR treatment has no proven clinically beneficial effect on those with PTSD type 1 who are of 'the wrong' genotype, has no proven clinically beneficial effect on those with only PTSD type 2, and has no clinically proven beneficial effect on any other mental or physical disorder.

In Chapter Eight, there is an abductively reasoned and plausibly inferred mechanism for the abnormal neurobiology of PTSD type 1 and its dependence on aspects of the person's genomics, and the genomic mechanism of the curative action of EMDR treatment. For those with PTSD type 1 who cannot respond to EMDR treatment, they can be greatly helped by Exposure Therapy, with or without adjunctive anti-anxiety substances.

PTSD type 2 is a 'generic dimensional disorder', i.e. not different in form from most other anxiety disorders. 'Dimensional' is defined as 'having sufficient depth and substance to be believable'. PTSD type 2 is characterised by having been caused by one or more experiences of mentally traumatic anxiety, giving rise to persisting anxiety and anxiety-related symptoms together with impairment in multiple areas of life over a significant period of time. It has no specific pattern for its many and varied non-specific anxiety-related symptoms. It has no recurrent abnormal-in-form flashbacks. It has no persistent peripheral oscillopsia on testing. It can have severely distressing-on-recall memories, that are normal-in-form memories, of the mental trauma or traumas that caused the anxiety disorder PTSD type 2.

From person to person, PTSD type 2 has a spectrum of severity ranging from severe to virtually 'clinically insignificant', i.e. present but virtually un-noticed until attention is drawn to it, and just believable. It can resolve spontaneously over time by merging imperceptibly with normal day-to-day anxiousness, but does not always, depending on current circumstances. Other than having followed mental trauma, it is similar in form to other generic anxiety disorders. The nature of the experiences of mentally traumatic stress can have been a mental shock, i.e. a sudden surge of high anxiety as with PTSD type 1, or less sudden, non-specific mentally traumatic stressors from one or more frightening or otherwise distressing mentally traumatic events. The nature of the causal traumatic event or events is immaterial. The time of onset of the symptoms may coincide with the time of the traumatic event(s) or develop some short time, a day or two, later.

PTSD type 2 has, just as PTSD type 1 can have, one or more non-specific anxiety-related symptoms. These can include nightmares, hyper-vigilance, exaggerated startle response, avoidance of external reminders, avoidance of thoughts and feelings associated with the traumatic event, headaches, inattentiveness, insomnia, emotional withdrawal, depressed mood, recurrent distressing, intrusive memories in normal form, episodic dissociation, episodic derealization, panic attacks . . .

PTSD type 2 can be diagnosed in anyone old enough to demonstrate persisting anxiety known to have followed significant recently experienced mental trauma.

PTSD type 2 can resolve spontaneously over time. EMDR treatment has no effect at all on PTSD type 2. PTSD type 2 cannot always spontaneously resolve if there is persisting traumatic stress from persisting traumatising events and or persisting mentally traumatising physical and or social circumstances (we come to so-called Complex PTSD just below). The resolution of PTSD type 2 can be helped along with Exposure Therapy with or without adjuvant anti-anxiety substances. There are no known genomic aspects to PTSD type 2.

PTSD type 2 can be present together with other mental disorders, including PTSD type 1, with personality disorders, with psychotic disorders, and together with physical disorders, including traumatic brain injury.

PTSD type 2 can persist indefinitely if there are indefinitely persisting stressors such as indefinitely persisting severe physical disability, severe persisting pain, and severe persisting psycho-social and or socio-economic threats.

From this above, it is clear that PTSD type 1 and PTSD type 2 can appear superficially virtually indistinguishable clinically. The

Visual Test is sensitive, reliable, and specific for the presence or absence of persistent peripheral oscillopsia and hence a sensitive, reliable, and specific test for the presence or absence of persistently recurrent normal flashbacks; and hence, a sensitive, reliable, and specific test for the presence of absence of PTSD type 1.

Attempting to detect the presence or absence of PTSD type 1 solely by detecting the presence or absence of one or more different forms of recurrent abnormal-in-form flashback memories is less clear-cut than using the Visual Test, and is mostly unnecessary. When PTSD type 1 and PTSD type 2 are present together, or either is present with one or more other mental disorders, the successful treatment of one form of PTSD will leave the other form of PTSD and or other mental disorder(s) still present.

Experiencing a mental shock, intense or otherwise, is not uncommon for anyone. And not all mental shocks are damaging. Most are briefly emotionally hurtful but do not amount to a mental disorder and can sooner or later be brushed off.

So-called Complex PTSD.

William of Ockham can be assured that Complex PTSD is not a third form of PTSD—-there is no plurality beyond a PTSD type 1 and a PTSD type 2. So-called Complex PTSD is not a unique clinical entity, as are PTSD type 1 and PTSD type 2. Complex PTSD is the clinical name given to an accumulation over the long term of personality disorder features engendered by repeated and prolonged mental trauma of PTSD type 1 and or PTSD type 2, i.e. it becomes a non-specific 'Post-traumatic Stress Personality Disorder', possibly combined with recurrent abnormal flashbacks and persistent peripheral oscillopsia of PTSD type 1. To have PTSD type 1 and PTSD type 2 properly recognised in the Complex PTSD collection of symptoms is very important. The confusion is that the term Complex PTSD could be applied to just about everyone with a PTSD type 1 and or a PTSD type 2 whose personality has any shortcomings that can possibly be related to their PTSD type 1 and or PTSD type 2. Anyone with PTSD type 1 and or PTSD type 2 from any cause and who suffers noticeable anxiety-related symptoms and or emotional outbursts can claim to have Complex PTSD, thereby devaluing the 'currency' of those with severe Complex PTSD and profound personality difficulties—the Complex PTSD of first responders following multiple untreated mental traumas, of refugees following hideous long-drawn-out torture, of long-term sex and other slavery, of mental and physical exploitation over many years . . .

The WHO criteria for Complex PTSD are, *in effect*, a 'persisting PTSD type 1 and or PTSD type2 together with the features of a personality disorder, a disorder with clinical features akin to so-called 'Borderline Personality Disorder'. The 'personality' symptoms include so-called 'disturbances of self-organisation, symptoms that can be defined as emotional dysregulation, interpersonal difficulties, and negative self-concept'.

The WHO criteria for 'PTSD' are simple: 're-experiencing a traumatic event in intrusions, flashbacks or nightmares; avoiding trauma-associated contexts and triggers; hypervigilance.'

This WHO clinically non-rigorous optional triad of symptoms for a 'PTSD' certainly does not differentiate between PTSD type 1 and PTSD type 2, a differentiation necessary when it comes to trial treatment with EMDR and when it comes to a description of Complex PTSD. Not all Complex PTSD cases have or have had PTSD type 1, and presumably not those cases for whom the childhood trauma occurred under the age of five. The clinical evidence strongly suggests that PTSD type 1 and/or PTSD type 2 can occur in people with or without a prior personality disorder and, with or without any other prior disorder, and with or without the genome for ADHD impairments (See later for the special relationship between PTSD type 1 and ADHD.)

Clinical features of the complex post-traumatic stress personality disorder, so-called Complex PTSD.

C-PTSD followed multiple situations, each giving PTSD type 2, with or without one or multiple situations, each giving an extra module of PTSD type 1.

C-PTSD symptoms include disturbances of self-organisation symptoms defined as emotional dysregulation, interpersonal difficulties, and negative self-concept, and can include recurrent abnormal re-experiencing memory flashbacks characteristic of PTSD type 1.

C-PTSD usually follows, but not necessarily, long, drawn-out trauma over months, years, or decades.

C-PTSD usually follows, but not necessarily, childhood trauma.

C-PTSD usually follows, but not necessarily, interpersonal trauma.

C-PTSD can frequently follow the mental traumas of long-lasting childhood abuse, childhood abandonment, long-lasting relationship abuse, sexual slavery, living for a long time as a refugee, living for a long time with long-lasting combat, or being deliberately and repeatedly tortured.

C-PTSD can follow multiple modules of PTSD type 1 from multiple traumatic mental shocks of long-serving first responders: firefighters, police officers, paramedics, combat service personnel . . . of either gender and older than adolescence.

Hopefully, concentrating on the 'personality' aspects of Complex PTSD, won't deflect focus from looking for, recognising, treating, and curing, if possible, co-occurring PTSD type 1 and PTSD type 2.

The end result of all adult personality development is determined mostly by luck, starting with the inheritance of good or not-so-good genes, followed by good or not-so-good life experiences from earliest childhood onwards to early adulthood. There are few people who have never experienced stressful mental trauma of one form or another while growing up, and there are few people with perfect personalities in the eyes of those who know them well.

PTSD type 1 and or PTSD type 2 or Complex PTSD can be

present together with a schizophrenic illness or a bipolar illness—though not always a priority for treatment. There are few mental or physical illnesses or injuries that could not be present at the same time. Rarely, Complex PTSD can resolve spontaneously over time, over decades.

The philosopher Karl Popper, who died in 1984, pointed out: 'being uncritical allows one to always find what is wanted to be found to confirm a theory'. The opposite also applies; fear of cognitive dissonance allows one to avoid finding anything that refutes one's own theory. Cognitive dissonance is a feeling of emotional discomfort from having to believe in two different things that one feels cannot both be right. Anyone involved with what they think might be PTSD type 1 may or may not want to find peripheral oscillopsia or a recurrent abnormal flashback memory, if asked to look for them. It has always been up to 'them' to tell 'us' what 'they' observe. All of this is called 'clinical science'; it is what the essence of this book relies upon.

FORMAL DEFINITION AND CLINICAL CRITERIA FOR PTSD Type 1

1. **PTSD type 1** has one necessary condition: it was caused by, and only by, and at the moment of, an experience of mental shock (the experience of a sudden surge of intense anxiety). The cause or severity of the mental shock is immaterial.

2. **PTSD type 1** is a categorical anxiety disorder. From the onset, it has one necessary-and-sufficient condition: a unique combined symptom of two invariant (never changing in form) and inseparable (impossible to disentangle or separate) unique clinical symptoms: (i) a unique abnormality of vision—persistent peripheral oscillopsia (as defined); (ii) one or more uniquely abnormal-in-form recurrent experiential (re-experiencing) flashback memories (as defined), each flashback memory being of one or more aspects of the emotional physical and or sensorial experiences

that were contemporaneous with the circumscribed moment of a mental shock, a sudden surge of intense anxiety, that caused the disorder, and further mental shocks that caused subsequent additional abnormally formed memories of subsequent sudden surges of intense anxiety. A combined complex-double-symptom forms one module of PTSD type 1; hence, there may be more than one module present from more than one circumscribed moment of mental shock at a previous or a subsequent time.

3. **PTSD type 1** has dimensional severity: from person to person. The spectrum of the subjective severity of its two invariant and inseparably linked symptoms is from severe and obtrusive to non-severe, unobtrusive, and virtually 'clinically insignificant'; the spectrum of the subjective severity of any associated non-specific anxiety-related symptoms is from severe to non-severe, to virtually 'clinically insignificant'; the spectrum of the objective dimension of severity of the non-specific event that engendered the mental shock ranges from large to small.

4. **PTSD type 1** can have non-specific anxiety-related symptoms. These include nightmares, hyper-vigilance, exaggerated startle response, avoidance of external reminders of the causal event, avoidance of thoughts and feelings associated with the causal event, headaches, inattentiveness, insomnia, emotional withdrawal, depressed mood, recurrent distressing, intrusive memories in normal form, episodic dissociation, episodic derealization, panic attacks.

5. **PTSD type 1** has non-specific anxiety-related symptoms common to PTSD type 2.

6. **PTSD type 1** cannot resolve spontaneously over time.

7. **PTSD type 1** is unlikely to be diagnoseable below the age of 5 years.

FORMAL DEFINITION AND CLINICAL CRITERIA OF PTSD Type 2

1. **PTSD type 2** is a dimensional, non-specific, generic anxiety disorder having no unique clinical features.

2. **PTSD type 2** has a necessary condition of having been caused by the experience of one or more mentally traumatic events, with or without mental shock. Its onset may be sudden, slow, or delayed for several days or longer.

3. **PTSD type 2** is a disorder of persisting anxiety and non-specific anxiety-related symptoms. The symptoms can include nightmares, hyper-vigilance, exaggerated startle response, avoidance of external reminders, avoidance of thoughts and feelings associated with the traumatic event, headaches, inattentiveness, insomnia, emotional withdrawal, depressed mood, recurrent distressing, intrusive memories in normal form, episodic dissociation, episodic derealization, panic attacks. These nonspecific amorphous symptoms of anxiety and distress can be in common with the same anxiety-related symptoms of PTSD type 1.

4. **PTSD type 2** has no unique, abnormal features of vision and no abnormal forms of memory recall but may have distressing, intrusive memories of normal form.

5. **PTSD type 2** has dimensional severity: the spectrum of the severity of any of its non-specific anxiety-related symptoms is from severe to un-noticed until attention is drawn; the spectrum of the objective dimension of the non-specific type of event that engendered the mental shock ranges from large to small, to being just clinically significant.

6. **PTSD type 2** can resolve spontaneously over time but not always does, depending on current or persisting mentally traumatic circumstances.

7. **PTSD type 2** has non-specific anxiety-related symptoms common to PTSD type 1.

8. **PTSD type 2** has no known age at which PTSD type 2 cannot occur, and it must be presumed that PTSD type 2 can arise at any age.

Post Traumatic Blast Disorder (PTBD)

When an experience of a mentally traumatic event is in the form of the exposure to an explosion and its blast wave - the propagation of a supersonic pressure gradient - then the impact of this is a blunt head injury, a Traumatic Brain Injury (a TBI), whether or not the experience also causes a PTSD type 1 and or a PTSD type 2. This TBI can be of any severity---with blast wave-related compressions and shearings of the brain tissues -giving micro- and macro-brain haemorrhages, and diffuse brain nerve cell axon injuries, all with short or long-term diverse effects, each virtually recoverable or virtually irrevocable.

With experiences of multiple blasts - gunshots, bomb blasts, shell blasts (whether the person is at the sending or receiving end) the long-term effects can be that of any oft-repeated TBIs (seen in boxers, contact field sport players, even in late-age brain atrophy) i.e., a widened third ventricle seen on brain imaging. Combat veterans and bombed-out civilians, with the double diagnosis of PTSD type 1 and or PTSD type 2 plus PTBD, are probably most noticeable *en masse* in combat veterans and collateral refugees. There is no specific active treatment for Post Traumatic Blast Disorder, PTBD (except in extreme cases of brain swelling where induced coma in a specialised unit may be used).

CHAPTER SIX

A schoolteacher's account of his own PTSD type 1.

Michael was referred to me, the psychiatrist, in 1980. Michael had been involved in a road accident in 1977 and complained he was still suffering from 'something' because of it. He was twenty-five at the time of the accident. He gave me his account of the accident:

While cycling to work on a rainy morning, he had, he was told later, collided with a truck, was knocked unconscious, and came to a few minutes later lying underneath the truck. He was totally unaware of what had happened to him when he came to. His retrograde amnesia was a result of a blow to his head and had left him with no memory of the accident a few minutes earlier or any memory of the few minutes before that. He could remember leaving home in the rain on his bicycle, but nothing further until after he came to.

He said that on first coming to, he had been totally bewildered. As he looked around, taking in the bewildering situation, he suddenly panicked and experienced a sudden surge of extreme anxiety. Inexplicably, he was under a truck, lying on a soaking wet road, unable to move, seeing blood and a bone sticking out from his trousers, seeing his leg was broken, and aware of the sound of pouring rain and of people shouting. Ten minutes later, he said, and after the worst of his panic had subsided, he had been gently pulled from under the truck. After a further ten minutes, an ambulance arrived, and he was off to the hospital. He eventually made a good physical recovery from his head injury and his broken leg, and he eventually returned to work five weeks later.

He was referred to me three years after the accident. Although he was back at work, he was by no means 'back to normal'. His wife had accompanied him to the psychiatric consultation, and she wanted her to say: "Michael has gone from being an active and jolly husband, father, and schoolteacher to how he was when he came out of hospital, which was how he still is now, with no improvement over three years. He prefers to sit in a corner, virtually a vegetable, emotionally cold, distant, irritable, cranky, and inattentive. He is ignoring his friends, becoming more and more reclusive and intolerant with the children at home and at school, and only just holding his temper, his knuckles going white when he is crossed. And saying almost every day, 'There's something wrong inside my head'. He has constantly recurring headaches, cannot concentrate normally, cannot get off to sleep at night for hours, and he has horribly panicky nightmares about anything and everything panicky".

Michael said the nightmares could wake him with a start and as often as not, he was then straight into the worst thing, the same panicky flashbacking-back memory, always the same, always re-experiencing, re-living that moment of panic after regaining consciousness and finding himself lying helpless under a truck. The same flashbacks could also come during the day. The flashbacks were getting no better; he was getting no better. His children were getting older. The family was losing heart. Could the psychiatrist help him?

He could not talk of his flashbacks without emotional upset. Whenever describing them, he was inevitably having an anxiety-packed flashing-back memory: visibly wet palms and forehead, visibly shaking, repeatedly clenching his fists. The flashback could be there immediately after waking from a nightmare or come at any time during the day; suddenly, he was panicky and could see everything exactly how it had been three years ago. It was as though there had been a video camera in his head at the moments of panic, and since then, it has been repeatedly replaying the scene of those moments. The scene, the 'picture', was a clear-as-a-bell, in full colour and transparent 're-playing video clip' of those moments. He was re-seeing the whole scene and re-experiencing the feeling of still lying there wet, panicky and in pain, bewilderingly trapped below a truck and looking bewilderingly at what was around him, fearing the worst.

Whether he had the flashback in the dark or in daylight, there was the bright red of the car on the other side of the road with rain pounding on it, just as bright red as it was—nothing special about that red car, but it just happened to have been noticed when looking from under the truck; the bone sticking out from his torn trouser leg was just as white, the blood just as red, the beige of the onlookers' raincoats was just as beige, their black umbrellas just as black. He could hear the rain as it had been, not just remember the sound of it, and hear the same words of the onlookers peering at him shouting "rescue" and "ambulance" as clear as he could hear his own voice telling of it; the pain in his leg the same as when he first came-to; the smell of the diesel was as though there was diesel in the room where he was having the flashback. Sometimes, a flashback would persist for a quarter of a minute, sometimes for five minutes or more. He would try to get it to go away by shaking his head, quickly opening and closing his eyes, pinching himself, getting up and leaving the room. If it were the middle of the night, then going downstairs to pace about, perhaps bang the table, hit the wall, have a whisky. . .. He could bring on the flashbacks if he was careless about his thinking, or they could be triggered by something on television. Mostly, the flashbacks came at any time and without reason. It was impossible to get back to sleep after one: his wife would go and sleep in the children's room to get herself back to sleep. With a flashback at school, he would excuse himself and walk out of the classroom until it had passed.

He had other intrusive and distressing memories flashing back, memories that were not part of the moments lying under the truck, not flashing back in the same vivid and panicky way as the flashbacks of that moment under the truck. These distressing, intrusive memories and dreams took him back to other unpleasant moments, memories that made him feel angry, depressed and humiliated memories of screaming with the pain in his leg as he was being pulled from underneath the truck by the helpful onlookers before the ambulance arrived. With those memories, there was no return of pain; it was just embarrassment. The same is true with the memory of waking from the anaesthetic in the hospital, seeing his plastered leg with weights attached, totally immobilising him in bed, and complaining angrily to the nurse when she tried to help him become more comfortable. Worst of all, remembering as a schoolboy arriving home from school and being told his father had been killed in an accident at work. When asked, he said he could certainly tell the difference between the very emotionally painful, normal-in-form flashing back memories and his very, very emotionally and physically painful obviously abnormal-in-form flashback memory.

There was little help I, the psychiatrist, could give to Michael. Michael had a PTSD type 1. Traumatic Neurosis had just been renamed to PTSD in that year, 1980. Michael had talked many times to psychologists, had taken anti-anxiety and anti-depressant medication from his doctor, and had waited to see if things would improve, but all to no avail.

I asked Michael to cooperate with the simple Visual Test. Michael and his wife were sceptical; he had had ink-blot tests and the likes from one psychologist, thinking Michael might be neurotic from childhood traumas and wanting to talk about the death of his father. One psychologist suspected a persisting post-concussion syndrome from brain-impact damage from the accident. Skull x-rays and brain CAT scans had shown nothing. There was nothing to suggest he had ADHD.

The simple Visual Test went ahead. Michael had persistent peripheral oscillopsia. This was of no concern to Michael or his wife since whatever it meant to the psychiatrist; it did not noticeably affect Michael. His wife asked to have the same quick, simple Visual Test. His wife had no persistent peripheral oscillopsia.

I asked to see Michael again, to follow him up every three to six months, and to repeat the simple eye test each time. Michael was followed up for ten years, and nothing changed—his general demeanour, the detailed nature of the abnormal flashbacks, and the persistent peripheral oscillopsia persisted unchanged.

Michael's story of his abnormal flashbacks was one of many similar stories of many people I had collected over those three years with Traumatic Neurosis, what had just been called PTSD. I could do nothing that was clinically effective for Michael or for any others—talk to them, yes, but nothing effective in the long term. For Michael, some short-lived help from this or that medication. Little at all from talking about the accident. Nothing until one day in 1990.

CHAPTER SEVEN

The investigation's 'necessary' clinical experiment: a trial of EMDR. Providing transformational evidentiary clinical findings about PTSD and experimental proof of the concept of EMDR.

In 1989, 'out of the blue', there came an anecdotal scientific paper describing the exceptional clinical observation of Dr Francine Shapiro, an American Psychologist. In 1989, Dr Shapiro published a paper, 'A new treatment for PTSD' * Her paper gave remarkable details of how she had unexpectedly and accidentally cured her own 'PTSD' (PTSD type 1, as we now know) whilst she was taking a walk in the park—and how the same peculiar technique had cured some others of their 'PTSD'.

*Shapiro, F. (1989). Eye movement desensitization and reprocessing: A new treatment for posttraumatic stress disorder. Journal of Behaviour Therapy and Experimental Psychiatry, 20, 211-217.

Dr Shapiro had been experiencing some distressing, anxiety-provoking, and constantly recurring, flashing-back 'pictures' of a very frightening traumatic event in the recent past. The recurring flashing-back pictures of the moment of mental shock, engendered by the event, were stubbornly, repeatedly distressing her, causing constant anxiety. To her surprise, the 'pictures' suddenly went away and never returned after she tried to get rid of the 'picture' by moving both her eyes rapidly and repeatedly from side to side while the 'picture' was there. Not only could she no longer get the pictures back after performing these side-to-side-eye movements—merely thinking about them would have certainly brought them back—but she could not bring back the extra anxiety she had always experienced with the recurring abnormal flashbacks. She could certainly remember the particularly distressing mentally traumatic event, and remember details of the recurring 'picture', but she could now remember them only normally, certainly somewhat distressingly, but without the 'picture', without re-living the panicky feelings, and without it suddenly appearing at random. The abnormal form of memory of that mentally traumatic event had been, she said, somehow 'reprocessed' into a normal form of memory. Dr Shapiro certainly knew first-hand what a post-traumatic stress disorder was for her, and hers was now, and unexpectedly, 'cured', gone for good. This was certainly an exceptional clinical observation. This was *an exception* she certainly treasured.

Dr Shapiro had several clients in her own psychological practice over the years, clients with similar anxiety-creating flashing back pictures of frightening events in the past—clients with one or other form of 'PTSD' whom she had been unable to help in any such dramatic a way as this. She had no idea how or why her side-to-side eye movements had worked. Undeterred, she wasted no time. Getting her private practice clients to re-enact her own scene-in-the-park eye movements had the same amazingly successful results. Dr Shapiro was curing 'PTSD'. She called her treatment 'Eye Movement Desensitisation and Reprocessing', now universally called EMDR.

To treat her clients, they merely had to sit comfortably in a chair, facing her. They were first asked to voluntarily re-evoke one of their abnormal re-experiencing flashbacks—a picture, a sensation, a sound—whatever comes. Then, holding their head still, they were asked to follow Dr Shapiro's fingers with their eyes as Dr Shapiro moved her hand in front of them, moving from far right to far left at about one to two cycles per second. The clients were to stop moving their eyes once the picture, sensation, sound, or whatever had gone. This run of side-to-side eye movements was repeated, perhaps several times, the clients re-evoking the picture etc. each time, until eventually the clients' pictures, etc. had gone, and the clients could not re-evoke any part of the abnormal re-experiencing flashback, despite trying.

What Dr Shapiro had published in her paper was 'epistemologically acceptable mechanistic reasoning', meaning what she was saying was acceptable to the philosophy of the theory of knowledge: that performing EMDR in the presence of an evoked recurrent abnormal re-experiencing memory of a traumatic experience, had a probability of causing a permanent conversion of that memory to normal form. In other words, the justification for the practice of EMDR treatment trials for those with a PTSD (only a PTSD type 1, it eventually turned out) was based on irrefutable, replicable, evidentiary clinical findings.

But, for most academic-minded psychiatrists at the time, her published paper was 'too anecdotal' and its content 'too counter-intuitive' and 'too psychological and not psychiatric' for them to give it a second thought. The majority of psychiatrists ignored its content. (Cesare Cremonini refused to look through Galileo's telescope—the simple device of not looking, and so able to ignore seeing, anything that does not fit with one's theory). Dr Shapiro's 'mistake and triumph' was to have tried to give the impression she had cured PTSD when, even in 1990, there was no generally acceptable clinical definition of exactly what 'PTSD' was for everyone to go by, and it was soon apparent that her EMDR wasn't always an effective treatment for everyone with the sort of PTSD that Dr Shapiro had cured for herself.

There are many things Dr Shapiro probably did not know about 'PTSD' at the time: life is not quite so simple for all with 'PTSD' as it appeared to be for Dr Shapiro when she cured her own 'PTSD' in the park. Nevertheless, her serendipitous discovery and her dissemination of the details of her discovery have been highly beneficial for very many thousands of people. Sadly, Dr Shapiro died in June 2019.

Details of how anyone can properly perform EMDR for PTSD for anyone over five or six years old are in Chapter Eleven. The chapters before Chapter Eleven should be read before trying EMDR. Sadly, properly performed EMDR does not work for everyone with 'PTSD', regardless of who properly performs the EMDR. And there is now a lot more to know about 'PTSD' before anyone should be trying EMDR on anyone.

Having read Dr Shapiro's paper in 1990, I immediately contacted Michael to make an appointment for a trial of this new treatment. The Editor of the journal in which EMDR was published was a good friend of Dr Shapiro: she had added her own quip to the readers of the article: "EMDR really does work; you should try it". Sceptical as Michael and his wife were, after ten years of being followed up, and no change at all in his PTSD for thirteen years, they felt Michael had nothing to lose. Before the treatment started, he was re-checked both for persistent peripheral oscillopsia and for the persisting presence of his abnormal re-experiencing flashback. Both had always remained unchanged from when Michael was first seen ten years before and thirteen years since the accident that had caused it.

This was to be the crucial experiment: what happens to persistent peripheral oscillopsia when subjected to EMDR treatment?

The neuropsychiatric, neuro-psychological experiment.

Michael's EMDR treatment continued for thirty minutes. It consisted of several runs of ten or so one-to-two-per-second side-to-side eye movements—rapid eye movements between fixed points are called **saccade**s. Michael's 'picture' kept going after each run of saccades, but he could still re-evoke the picture after each run. But he said he noticed after each run of saccades the picture came back with less detail—the red-in-colour car was, run by run, a duskier red; the outlines of the car becoming blurred; the voices becoming distant and indistinct; the noise of the rain becoming less clear; the pain in his leg becoming less; the picture of the bone sticking out slowly faded and now gone altogether. This appeared to suggest the abnormally formed memory engram was being processed, step-by-step, to a normal, non-re-experiencing form of memory engram. After every few runs of saccades, his vision was re-tested for persistent peripheral oscillopsia, and each time, he reported that the oscillations were still there, but the oscillations were definitely decreasing in amplitude. This appeared to suggest that persistent peripheral oscillopsia was also decreasing step-by-step, doing so in step with the normalising memory engram. The two uniquely abnormal symptoms of PTSD type 1 were maintaining the 'pattern' of staying together as a module, even as they were being eliminated step-by-step and in step, still together to the end.

At the end of half an hour of EMDR treatment, after eleven or twelve runs of saccades, Michael said that for the first time since the accident thirteen years before, he was quite unable to evoke any detail at all of the abnormal memory engrams of the re-experiencing flashback. And the anxiety was gone. At the end of that half hour of EMDR treatment, the Visual Test for oscillopsia was negative: Michael could discern no hint of apparent movement in the periphery. Seemingly, his PTSD type 1 had been cured there and then—by thirty minutes of simple non-invasive treatment after thirteen years of unchanging PTSD: the abnormally formed memory engram of the happenings experienced during that moment of panic had reformed to a normal form of memory engram of the happenings experienced during that moment of panic. And the abnormal peripheral oscillopsia had returned to stable vision. The anxiety level had reduced to a normal, unobtrusive level. This man's PTSD type 1 had been permanently cured by Dr Shapiro's EMDR, just as she said it would be. But! . . . we come to the 'buts' very shortly.

This treatment result of Michael provided a transformational evidentiary clinical finding—one of many to come.

The first piece of transformational clinical evidence is that there is an abnormal compound-clinical-symptom having two invariants (always unchanging and there together) different abnormal clinical phenomena: (i), persistent peripheral oscillopsia, and (ii), an abnormally formed memory that is, on recurrent recall, an emotional, physical and sensorial re-experiencing of the emotional, physical and sensorial experiences consciously noticed and remembered during a moment of a sudden surge of intensely high anxiety. If (i) is present then (ii) is present—(i) and (ii) come together, stay together, and go together simultaneously. The two symptoms are inseparably linked. This unique compound symptom appears to be unique to that form of PTSD type 1 with which Michael and many others had presented.

The second piece of transformational clinical evidence is that properly performed EMDR treatment can permanently cure some people with that form of PTSD type 1.

Very soon after the success of Michael's EMDR treatment, there were many such evidentiary clinical findings to confirm that properly performed EMDR treatment cannot permanently cure all people with a clinical presentation of PTSD type 1 that is identical to the clinical presentation of Michael's PTSD type 1.

Amongst the people who presented to the investigation, there were evidentiary clinical findings that the effectiveness and success of EMDR treatment for those presenting with PTSD type 1, depends on many factors, the most significant of which appears to be the genotype of the person with PTSD type 1. It appeared that those with PTSD type 1 of the phenotype of blue eyes, light skin, and fair hair were far more likely to respond successfully to EMDR treatment than those with PTSD type 1 of the phenotype of dark eyes, olive-coloured skin, and dark hair.

There were evidentiary clinical findings that properly performed EMDR treatment cannot cure any other mental or physical disorder, including the one other form of 'PTSD', PTSD type 2. We comment further on genomic factors of PTSD type 1 in Chapter Eight.

No, schoolteacher Michael was not quite fully cured of all aspects of the post-mental-trauma mental difficulties of having had post-traumatic stress disorder for thirteen years. He was overjoyed in one way—getting rid of the flashbacks and most of the anxiety. He did not miss the persistent peripheral oscillopsia; he had only noticed it after visiting the psychiatrist and having The Visual Test. He was still seriously lacking in self-esteem and self-confidence, not bouncing straight back to exactly how he had been the day before the accident. It took a lot more than half an hour for all the consequences of having post-traumatic stress disorder type 1 for thirteen years to become as socially, psychologically, and intellectually well as he was going to be. He was now thirty-eight.

Michael and his wife were followed up. After a year, his demeanour was indistinguishable from that of any other self-confident, highly intelligent middle-aged schoolteacher, loving father of two now eighteen-year-old young adult children, and loving husband to his wife. Yes, he could remember all the events, but the memories seemed very distant, free from emotion, and still fading in detail. The accident seemed to be years and years ago. The only persisting worry was whether the PTSD would come back. He was assured that, in all probability, Michael would need another comparable mental shock from another comparable frightening experience for him to have PTSD again, and that was improbable. There were still memories of the other distressing events, but they were less bothersome and intrusive than they had been when he had the persisting anxiety of PTSD type 1.

Dr Shapiro eventually formed an EMDR International Association to which, for a fee, fellow psychologists could enrol, learn, and be 'certified to practice, EMDR'. I, Michael's psychiatrist, had tried EMDR treatment within five days of briefly reading her short paper. Five days after reading the paper, confirming it certainly was effective in eliminating PTSD type 1 for Michael. It seemed there was not a great deal to learn about. There is certainly a lot to learn about PTSD type 1 and PTSD type 2: when to do EMDR, and for whom. Dr Shapiro was contacted by phone to let her know about persistent peripheral oscillopsia, and how it was eliminated simultaneously by EMDR. By then, Dr Shapiro was terribly busy building her credibility and publicising EMDR around the world. Under-standably, Dr Shapiro was too busy to take notice of odd news coming from someone she had never heard of, telling of something both counter-intuitive and too insignificant to merit her attention.

It had soon become evident, as just above, that when EMDR was tried on many people with PTSD type 1, the EMDR was far from always successful, but it was gratifyingly successful for many. For some with PTSD type 1 it had, inexplicably, no effect—no treatment response at all, no matter how many runs of saccades of how many different sessions on how many different days.

There were some readily understandable reasons why EMDR failed for some people. Some with PTSD type 2, as per the clinical criteria given above, EMDR did nothing. For many with PTSD type 1, being asked to voluntarily evoke an abnormal flashback was so anxiety-provoking that it was more than they could tolerate. For some with PTSD type 1 there were too many abnormal flashbacks from too many frightening moments from experiencing too many traumatic events. For them, no abnormal flashback would remain in focus long enough before being replaced by another flashing. EMDR, when it was effective, was only effective for people with recurrent abnormal flashbacks and associated persistent peripheral oscillopsia. Many with PTSD type 2 had high anxiety and horri-fying memories that were distressing memories coming back in a quite normal, non-experiential form and not accompanied by per-sistent peripheral oscillopsia on testing: for them, EMDR had no effect at all, no matter how thoroughly EMDR was performed and re-performed. But there were many inexplicable failures for people with a PTSD type 1 indistinguishable from Michael's PTSD type 1 and others the same—but they were people of a distinctly different phenotype from Michael.

Why did EMDR work when it worked? Why did EMDR not work when it appeared that it should? Chapter Eight gives some evidentiary clinical findings and the most plausible and reasonable inferences that can be taken from them on what could be 'going on' in the brain with PTSD type 1 and what, how and why with successful EMDR treatment.

EMDR is still practised widely by many psychologists for many conditions seemingly unconnected with any form of PTSD. Since EMDR undoubtedly did something dramatically good for some people with 'PTSD', and apparently for no good reason, it was reasonably thought by many that it might do something good for people with things other than 'PTSD'. It is hard to know what the "EMDR International Association" does without being a member of the Association. If there are beneficial effects for many of the people with many different uncomfortable mental states, and whether the beneficial effects are placebo effects or not, then all to the good for those for whom it gives subjective benefit. There appear to be no clinical tests to confirm its effectiveness for those being treated for something other than PTSD type 1, just the anecdotal subjective say-so of some of their clients, their clients happily paying for and getting what they wanted, i.e. deeming themselves to have been "cured". There are no treatment-emergent adverse events other than disappointment when nothing beneficial happens from trying EMDR treatment.

We must now ask: Can a mental shock (implying a sudden surge of intense anxiety) cause a PTSD type 1 with a persistently recurrent abnormal re-experiencing flashback and persistent peripheral oscillopsia on testing in some people, not in others? That one thing can follow another, that the two things correlate in time, does not imply that the first thing caused the second thing: correlation does not mean causation, and especially so when the first thing is not always followed by the second.

Professor Bradford Hill, a London, UK epidemiologist, whose 1950 hypothesis was that cigarette smoking 'causing' lung cancer, had to be clear on issues of 'cause and effect' in human epidemiology. He wrote a checklist (below) of nine criteria needing to be met before saying that a specific cause could be said to be related to a specific outcome. In the context of this book, how many criteria are met between a Mental Shock, and it being reasonably plausible to say it was the cause of a uniquely abnormal linked persistently recurrent abnormal flashback and persistent peripheral oscillopsia in some people, not in all people? Is it yes, no, or dubious? Here are Bradford Hill's nine criteria for 'a specific cause of a disorder to be acceptably plausible'. The *(Yes)* at the end of each means hopefully yes for Mental Shock being a cause of a PTSD type 1 (with persistently recurrent abnormal re-experiencing flashbacks and persistent peripheral oscillopsia) in some people, not in others.

1. Strength (effect size): A small association does not mean there is not a causal effect; the larger the association, the more likely it is causal. (*Yes*)

2. Consistency (reproducibility): Consistent findings observed by different people with different samples strengthen the likelihood of an effect. *(Yes)*.

3. Specificity: Causation is likely if there is a very specific population at a specific site and disease with no other likely explanation. The more specific an association between a factor and an effect is, the bigger the probability of a causal relationship. *(Yes)*

4. Temporality: The effect has to occur after the cause (and if there is an expected delay between the cause and expected effect, then the effect must occur after that delay). *(Yes)*

5. Biological gradient: Greater exposure should generally lead to a greater incidence of the effect. However, in some cases, the mere presence of the factor can trigger the effect. In other cases, an inverse proportion is observed: greater exposure leads to lower incidence. *(Yes)*

6. Plausibility: A plausible mechanism between cause and effect is helpful (but Hill noted that knowledge of the mechanism is limited by current knowledge). *(Yes)*

7. Coherence: Coherence between epidemiological and laboratory findings increases the likelihood of an effect. However, Hill noted that ". . . lack of such [laboratory] evidence cannot nullify the epidemiological effect on associations. . ." *(Yes)*.

8. Experiment: "Occasionally, it is possible to appeal to experimental evidence. Different people have very different susceptibilities in different circumstances to suffer evidence". *(Yes)*

9. Analogy: The effect of similar factors may need to be considered. *(Yes)*

Number six of the nine is the term 'biological plausibility', a relationship between any claim about a cause and an outcome that is consistent with existing biological and medical knowledge. Hill did note that knowledge of the claimed outcome might be limited by current knowledge. We have a way to go yet before we can comfortably come to Chapter Eight and the clinical evidence supporting a plausible mechanism consistent with current knowledge: a sudden momentary surge of anxiety, giving rise to an epigenetic insertion and a permanent PTSD type 1 in some people, not all people.

We saw in Chapter Two how Oppenheim had accepted intuitively the reality of some pathology, some 'real physical injury to the brain' in Traumatic Neurosis having been caused by 'fright'. Intuition is not quite enough— intuition may be true but not provable'. We are left with having to collect clinical evidence for the likelihood, never the certainty, of there being 'real physical injury to the brain in response to experiencing a mental shock'. Is just one sudden surge of anxiety enough to inflict permanent damage to the brain? It seems a little cause for a big effect, a sort of butterfly flapping its wings in Africa causing a hurricane in Texas.

The abnormal clinical phenomenon of a persistently recurrent abnormal flashback being inseparably linked to persistent peripheral oscillopsia is the pattern of an abnormal complex mental phenomenon: a uniquely abnormal form of a memory engram recall linked to a uniquely abnormal form of vision. Something had gone wrong in the brain of that person, at that moment of mental shock, to cause the brain to form an abnormal form of memory engram of the happenings over that same moment, and, at the same time, to permanently disrupt the stability of visual perception in the periphery of vision, and, to give rise to persisting anxiety. The evidence coming from the effects of successful EMDR treatment on the simultaneous elimination of the two unique symptoms, plus a simultaneous diminution in anxiety, further suggests a single cause. How and why? We come to the evidentiary clinical findings from which the most plausible inferences for 'how and why' in Chapter Eight. A mental shock appears to be the root cause of PTSD type 1 in some people, but not in people with PTSD type 2. In Chapter Eight, we cover a root cause analysis of the evidence for one form of PTSD that cannot spontaneously resolve, called PTSD type 1, and one form of PTSD, called PTSD type 2, that can but does not always spontaneously resolve.

CHAPTER EIGHT

The neurobiology of PTSD type 1:

Geneticists' most plausible and reasonable genomic inferences from their personal evidentiary clinical experiences.

Abductive reasoning is a form of logical inference. It starts with an observation or set of observations. In Part One of this Chapter, the observations are the evidentiary clinical findings that anyone can seek out and confirm. Together with the personal clinical experiences of two geneticists, unknown to each other, each with PTSD type 1 caused by the experience of a mental shock, and each having been permanently cured by successful EMDR treatment. Part Two of this Chapter seeks to find the simplest and most plausible inferences regarding the neurobiological mechanisms of their clinical experiences.

In philosophical Kantian terminology, it is speculating on the noumena, the unknowable reality, based on the known phenomena, i.e. speculating on the evidentiary clinical findings, and the known facts of genomics.

Part One of Chapter Eight. What we do know.

PTSD type 1 is complicated—virtually a 'Complex System'—with several interacting biological entities, two of them unique clinical entities.

Studies using all the usual neurological diagnostic tools, the ones of enormous help in neurological diagnosis and neurological research, giving us Electro-encephalography (EEG), Computerized Axial Tomography (CAT Scan), functional Magnetic Resonance Imaging (fMRI), and Positron-emission tomography (PET-scans), have all turned out to be of little or no help in diagnosis, useful research, or understanding of 'PTSD', let alone the two different PTSD type 1 and PTSD type 2. Much the same goes for research into the different chemical neurotransmitters and the human body's hormones in relation to PTSD type 1 and PTSD type 2.

The massive and expensive Magneto-encephalogram (MEG), however, can show an elevated production of focally generated slow waves of one to four cycles per second in those with a 'PTSD' compared with those people without a 'PTSD' The MEG detects the brief changes in magnetism secondary to brief electric currents. This suggests the likelihood of there being 'a central rhythm generator' responsible for the one to four cycles per second rhythmicity of the persistent peripheral oscillopsia of PTSD type 1. Obviously, more detailed research on this association is warranted, e.g., is the rhythm restricted to those with PTSD type 1? Does the rhythm frequency correlate with the oscillopsia frequency? Is it absent immediately following successful EMDR treatment that abolishes peripheral oscillopsia? The MEG is a large and somewhat cumbersome apparatus.

Inevitably, previous research has so far depended on 'PTSD' as defined by the clinically *ad hoc* criteria given in DSM or ICD, though, intuitively, it seems most likely that those with significant PTSD type 1 were more likely to have been selected for the most complicated and expensive investigations.

The anxiety levels with PTSD type 1 and PTSD type 2 vary from person to person, as they do with anyone with an anxiety disorder, and when anxiety levels are high, cerebral blood flow imaging techniques are likely to show changes indicating increased blood flow more in and around the right-sided amygdala nucleus than in the left. Other brain imaging studies have shown that the experience of traumatic events tend to 'activate' the right hemisphere of the brain and 'deactivate' the left side. PTSD. 'Symptom severity was positively related to regional cerebral blood flow in the right amygdala'.

Using bilateral implanted electrodes to electrically stimulate the amygdala nuclei in people with severe intractable 'combat PTSD' is said to have 'helped somewhat'. It is not a treatment likely to catch on. That it was used at all is an indication of just how desperately severe 'combat PTSD' can be.

The abductive reasoning we are coming to had not been aiming to pin-point any specific location in the brain for what has gone wrong in the brain in PTSD type 1, but as we are coming to, it can be reasonably inferred that there is a three-dimensional topographic site, meaning relating to the arrangement of the physical features of a specific location in the brain in which *three* constituent parts are functionally interrelated, i.e. an abnormally high anxiety, an abnormally formed engram memory of a mentally traumatic event, and an abnormal form of rhymical visual perception, the oscillopsia, of PTSD type 1. *How and where* do the saccades of EMDR treatment 'work' to simultaneously normalise the functioning of these *three* abnormalities in some people with a PTSD type 1, even if EMDR cannot do the same for others with a seemingly identical PTSD type 1 but being of a different phenotype?

At this stage, the best we can do to answer these questions is to abductively reason from a ***root cause analysis*** of the fully testable new evidentiary clinical findings, an explanation for a PTSD type 1 and a PTSD type 2. The first step in ***root cause analysis*** is to gather data, and clinical evidence. We have gathered the data. What is to follow is a list of the data collected, i.e. *the clinical observational consequences of the investigation*: a recapitulation of what we do know.

How the physicality, the objective reality, of a memory engram could be validly envisaged is beyond conceptual grasp—it is one of

Kant's *noumena* (the unknowables) — but intuitively talk about its subjective features we must.

So, just what is normal memory formation and recall? Well, a normally functioning brain, when in full consciousness, is aware of, notices, and experiences certain things that are happening. And, virtually contemporaneously, the brain is encoding (laying down) and storing memory engrams of those certain things that are happening, all experiences, that the brain is conscious of; this encoded information, the memory engram, can be recalled later. The highly complex hypothetical 'physical trace', the 'physicality' of the memory engram, intuitively involves (most likely) protein molecules in the chromosome of some of the brain's neurons concerned with memory. These processes are thought to be regulated by a gene protein called abrineurin, a 'Brain Derived Neurotropic Factor' (a BDNR). Once in storage, the *information detail* of the formed memory engram tends to fade away, bit by bit, over time. Some relatively 'unimportant' information detail fades away very quickly (a short-term memory), some 'more important' information detail 'never' fades away completely (a long-term memory)—and all are thought to be controlled by the gene protein, abrineurin. This sounds precise, but 'memory' as we know it is by no means always precise, all too often unreliable, unpredictable, and fickle.

It is reasonable to postulate that if some aspect of the brain's memory mechanism is functioning abnormally during a circumscribed moment of time, e.g., some aspect of the abrineurin protein is functioning abnormally, then the memory engram of the happenings, the experiences, during that circumscribed moment of time, could not have been fully encoded or encoded in abnormal form: either way, that engram is contemporaneously stored in abnormal form. A circumscribed 'moment in time' in this context is from a fraction of a second to two or so seconds, i.e. the 'duration of a mental shock', 'the time taken for a sudden surge of intense anxiety'. The abnormally formed memory engram, *can only be recalled as an abnormally formed memory engram of the happenings and expe-*

riences that were contemporaneously noticed and recorded during that circumscribed moment of mental shock. It is a rest-of-life permanent, long-term, abnormally formed, memory engram—it does not fade away bit by bit over time. We shall call this an abnormally formed memory engram—though unsure whether to intuit that this is the first stage of normal memory engram formation awaiting full processing, or whether it is a malformation of a memory engram, awaiting some form of repair back to a normal form: intuitively, the former seems the more likely.

(As we shall see just below, for some people with PTSD type 1, not all people with PTSD type 1, EMDR treatment has the ability to convert that incompletely or abnormally formed engram to normal form.)

In PTSD type 1, there is more than just the abnormally stored and abnormally recalled engram; there is also an abnormal persistent experience of *high anxiety persisting from that moment,* and *persistent peripheral oscillopsia persisting from that moment* — all three persisting from that moment. This persisting trio of abnormal clinical features constitutes 'one module of PTSD type 1'.

Transient anxiety is not unusual following a short-lived frightening experience. Transient wavy vision is not all that an unusual accompaniment of transient anxiety, e.g., of a panic attack. But a persisting abnormal form of recurring abnormally formed re-experiencing memory engram that is accompanied by both of these and all of the three persisting indefinitely together is spectacularly unique to PTSD type 1!

Successful properly performed EMDR treatment allows these three features to recover simultaneously, step-by-step and in-step, to a normal level of anxiety, a normal peripheral vision, and a normal-in-form memory engram of the happenings during that momentary surge of high anxiety, i.e., in the process, permanently eliminating one module of PTSD type 1.

In very few cases (exceptions), properly performed EMDR can totally and permanently cure and eliminate one module of PTSD type 1 within ten seconds of starting the first saccades—'exceptions that are treasured'.

Repeated, *un*successful properly performed EMDR leaves all three clinical features of PTSD type 1 unchanged for the rest of life.

Two academic geneticists from different universities were referred to me as clients (patients) at different times. The two geneticists never met each other or communicated with each other (as far as I know). One of the two geneticists had ADHD impairments also. Each had been referred by their different doctors for treatment of multi-modal PTSD type 1. They each had experienced sudden mental shocks—experiencing a sudden surge of intense anxiety—at the moment of onset of each of their PTSD type 1s. They each had experienced the features of their recurrent abnormal-in-form re-experiencing 'flashback' recalls of the memories of the moments of onset of each of their PTSD type 1s. They had each experienced persistent peripheral oscillopsia, they had each experienced persistent anxiety, they had each experienced these features from the moment of the events that caused their PTSD type 1s. Subsequently, they had each experienced the way that the abnormal memory, the abnormal vision, and the abnormal level of anxiety, were all permanently eliminated, step-by-step and in-step, with their multiple successful EMDR treatments.

They knew that properly performed EMDR was not successful for everyone with PTSD type 1.

They knew that anxiety can interfere with normal physiological functioning in many different ways, e.g., that anxiety can give rise to changes in the distribution of blood flow and blood pressure; to changes in heart and respiratory rate and rhythm; to irritability of bowel and bladder; to raised cortisol and adrenaline hormone secretions; to disruptions of short- and long-term immunological functioning; to all too-often-fatal sudden irregularities of heart rhythm with or without irrecoverable heart muscle damage—the potentially fatal 'Takotsubo cardiomyopathy' (this form of anxiety effect seemingly accounts for 'death from a broken heart' from the anxiety-ridden grief of mourning); they knew of the clinical evidence that an apparently spontaneous panic attack can provide the sudden surge of intense anxiety, the mental shock, to cause a PTSD type 1 in some people. In other words, they were each fully informed of the defining clinical characteristics of PTSD type 1 and PTSD type 2.

They knew high anxiety of a panic attack or near panic can give rise to transient subjective 'wavy vision', a form of transient irregular oscillopsia and subjective vestibular-type dizziness.

From the accounts of a few people with PTSD type 1 it *appears to them* the persisting oscillopsia was present from the moment of the sudden surge of anxiety. This could never be confirmed for all people seen with PTSD type 1. *Brief irregular oscillopsia*, 'wavy vision', sometimes experienced at moments of sudden high anxiety such as a panic attack, can occur in those with PTSD type 1 or PTSD type 2 as they can be with anyone without PTSD type 1 or PTSD type 2.

We know PTSD type 1 persists lifelong if not cured. We know PTSD type 2 can resolve spontaneously, but only in the absence of persisting or repeated adverse circumstances, for example, persisting PTSD type 2 in the often-life-long personality disorder of Complex PTSD.

We know for *some* people but not others, the repeated saccades (rapid side-to-side eye movements) of properly performed EMDR can, step-by-step, permanently eliminate the abnormally formed memory engram, replacing it with a normal memory engram, a normally formed memory, of the circumscribed moment of mental shock, and simultaneously permanently eliminate the peripheral oscillopsia and simultaneously permanently eliminate the anxiety. It can do this all *within ten seconds or less of starting the EMDR in a few exceptional cases of PTSD type 1.* We recall that in information theory, 'exceptions hold more information than non-exceptions'. At the other extreme, it may take many months of repeated EMDR treatment to eliminate a single module of PTSD type 1 and take somewhere in between those times in most cases of the successful EMDR treatment of PTSD type 1.

We know from evidentiary clinical findings collected from the later stages of the 30-year clinical investigation that people with the genome for ADHD impairments appear significantly more likely to develop PTSD type 1 in response to an experience of a mental shock, than are those without the genome for ADHD impairments. (See Chapter Nine for the evidentiary clinical findings of an association of PTSD type 1 and the genome for ADHD impairments.)

We know from the long-term evidentiary clinical findings of the 30-year investigation that certain people with PTSD type 1 who are of the phenotype dark-coloured hair and eyes and olive skin are far less likely to respond successfully to properly performed EMDR than those with PTSD type 1 who are of the phenotype light-coloured eyes and hair and light-coloured skin. The former have accounted for most of the unfortunate patients with EMDR-treatment-resistant PTSD type 1.

We know there are no evidentiary clinical findings that properly performed EMDR has demonstrable, provable clinical effects on people with other mental disorders, including PTSD type 2, or physical disorders, but perhaps, and only, has some 'clinically useful' placebo effects.

We know that there are four unique clinical features of PTSD type 1, features not occurring in any other mental or physical disorder: (i), the abnormal form of memory recall, (ii) persistent peripheral oscillopsia, (iii) the invariant joint presence of (i) and (ii), forming a module of PTSD type 1, and (iv), the response or non-response of PTSD type 1 to the unique treatment, 'properly performed EMDR', a success or failure mainly depending on the person's genotype.

PTSD type 1 has only been diagnosed in those over five years old or so. We have *not* seen any cases where confirmed PTSD type 1 appears to have arisen before the age of five years. But, we do not know what effect a mental shock can have on a child under the age of five years who has a phenotype known to be susceptible to mental trauma damage.

We know that most of the clinical observations spoken of here have been of Northern Europeans, some Southern Europeans, and Iberians, and not many of other ethnicities. We certainly have not seen a case of PTSD type 1 in persons from all countries, in persons of all ethnicities, and all genotypes.

There are increasing anecdotal reports that many people with PTSD, unspecified whether PTSD type 1, PTSD type 2 or both, can *appear to be* 'completely cured' by Exposure Therapy, some people with the adjunctive use of 'strictly controlled MDMA and psychotherapy'. It is not yet known whether, or if so, at what stage, the persistent peripheral oscillopsia of PTSD type 1, i.e. the complete module of PTSD type 1, can be eliminated by 'strictly controlled MDMA and exposure therapy psychotherapy', confirming or refuting a 'complete cure of PTSD type 1'. Hopefully, it soon will be known one way or another.

That is the data, the observational evidentiary clinical findings. Now to the abductive reasoning, reasoning beyond the data, beyond fact—the most plausible and reasonable inferences taken beyond what we know.

The virtual incomprehensible complexity of neurobiology did not deter either of the geneticists from inferring from their knowledge of all the above and their personal experiences, that only an ***epigenetic insertion*** could be the cause of each PTSD type 1 module, and successful EMDR treatment of each PTSD type 1 module could have been effected only by an ***epigenetic reversal*** for each PTSD type 1 module.

The inferences had been drawn from the two geneticists' personal knowledge as patients with multi-modular PTSD type 1 permanently cured by multiple sessions of EMDR, from their knowledge of everything written here learned during their many treatment sessions, and from their learning, research, and experiences as senior academic geneticists.

The two senior geneticists were each pleased to be rid of their PTSD type 1, and each pleased to retain their client anonymity.

Part Two of Chapter Eight.

In terms of present-day conceptual knowledge, what we can now plausibly and reasonably infer from what we now know.

To quote Thomas Huxley, the eighteenth-century scientist: "Anyone who is practically acquainted with scientific work is aware that those who refuse to go beyond fact rarely get as far as fact. Going beyond fact has a legitimate and potentially useful part to play in optimising the management of the problem". He was writing to Charles Darwin about Darwin's inferences on the origin of species taken from the biological findings from his investigations. He was stressing the part that intuition can play in scientific endeavour.

'A most plausibly probable neurobiology of PTSD type 1'.

What follows is not claimed to be *the* **ultimate cause of something**. It is not claimed to be the **Verae Cause of PTSD type 1**. However, to return to Huxley," Going beyond fact has a legitimate and potentially useful part to play in optimising the management of the problem".

A sudden surge of high anxiety of a momentary mental shock can instantly engender an epigenetic modification of some DNA molecules involved in the current 'virtual real time', contemporaneous, memory engram formation. The epigenetic modification involves epigenetic compounds, methyl-groups, (CH3), suddenly tagging themselves onto the molecules of some aspect of DNA, a process catalysed by the enzyme methyltransferase. Epigenetic modification entails modification of the functions or expressions of those DNA molecules. It is not a heritable modification; it is not a DNA mutation. Those DNA molecules engaged in the memory imprinting, the memory engram, of the contemporaneous happenings *during the moment* of the sudden surge of high anxiety, are tagged with one or more methyl groups.

The memory imprinting, the formation of the memory engram, of the contemporaneously experienced happenings during that moment of high anxiety by those methyl-tagged DNA molecules, is abnormal imprinting. Immediately after that circumscribed momentary surge of anxiety has passed, then *normal memory engram imprinting resumes*: further methyl group tagging does not occur. *The abnormally formed engram remains permanently in abnormal form*: the contents can only be recalled, not as a normal memory can be recalled i.e. as *an account*, but recalled as an abnormal flashing-back *re-experiencing* of the emotional, physical, and sensory experiences during that circumscribed moment of the surge of anxiety, the mental shock.

If the 'physical' (CH3 group) epigenetic insertion takes place in just one location, as one would intuit, one would suppose it is in the right-sided amygdala region. The corpus callosum—the thick band of fibres passing from one hemisphere to the other, bridging the third ventricle—will ensure some degree of integration between left and right, rather than there being a 'physical' (CH3 group) bilateral epigenetic insertion as one would not intuit.

For some people with PTSD type 1, not all properly performed EMDR treatment can bring about an apparent reversal of the epigenomic modifications of that DNA, by de-methylation of those tagged molecules of DNA. This allows the abnormally formed engram to be processed to a normal form of engram, a normal in form long-term memory, and at the same time, eliminating both the high anxiety and the peripheral oscillopsia of that module of PTSD type 1—one would have to intuit successful EMDR needing to be 'physically' (eliminating the CH3 group) effective on the right side only.

There is some speculation on just how EMDR does what it does for some people with PTSD type 1, but no speculation on why it does not do the same for other people with PTSD type 1. There is clinical evidence to plausibly infer that the success or failure of EMDR is dependent on the genotype, the genetic make-up, of the person with the PTSD type 1.

It is known that in the region of the right side of the brain where this abnormal form of memory engram is believed to be (in effect stored) and from where the anxiety is maintained (in or around the anterior insular cortex, closely connected with the amygdala nucleus) there is (in animals) an area of the cerebral cortex that can be electrically activated by movements seen in the visual fields: this is presumed to be part of the oculo-vestibular reflex system (to be described a few paragraphs below). In the anterior portions of the insular cortex, there is also a 'centre' for 'the emotion of 'disgust'. We know that a mental shock from either sudden disgust or sudden fear can engender PTSD type 1.

The insular cortex is the portion of the cerebral cortex that is enfolded between the temporal and parietal lobes, deep inside the lateral sulcus of each hemisphere. The insular cortex cannot be seen from the outside of the human brain and, hence, it is not easily approached for investigation with electrodes. There is multiple reciprocal neuronal interconnectivity between the oculo-vestibular portion of the posterior insular cortex and the very close-by amygdala nucleus—the nucleus that on the right side appears to be continually overactive in PTSD type 1, as judged by its continually increased regional blood flow on the right side, not on the left side. There are also the findings on magnetoencephalogram of 1 to 4 per second electrical impulses in those with a 'PTSD' — if a PTSD type 1, then those electrical impulses might correlate with the visual oscillations of peripheral oscillopsia before successful EMDR and absent after successful EMDR. It does not presently say just how localising these electrical impulses are seen to be.

The association between clinical increased anxiety, clinical persistent peripheral oscillopsia, and a clinical abnormally-formed memory engram of a mentally traumatic event, and the amygdala nucleus, suggests localised major neuronal interconnectivity on the right side of the brain, causing the two unique clinical manifestations of PTSD type 1. Hence, the right-sided insular cortex, deep inside the lateral sulcus of the right cerebral hemisphere, appears to be a brain hub, linking large-scale brain systems, and multimodal integration sites, which is believed to be 'how the brain works' in PTSD type 1: in our case the amygdala nucleus involved in memory and anxiety, and the ocular vestibular system involved in, amongst other things, reflex bilateral side-to-side eye movements in response to head movements. An epigenetic insertion into this right-sided integrative brain hub could permanently disturb its functioning. It seems that its collective normal functioning can be restored by EMDR, i.e. by connecting the evoked abnormal memory engram to multiple saccades—this appears to dislodge the CH3 methyl molecule, with the help of the enzyme demethylation transferase, *if the person's genome allows it*. So, is this 'where-and-how' successful multiple saccades EMDR treatment effective in curing PTSD type 1?

i.e. not forgetting the normal functioning of the oculo-vestibular reflex that ensures the eyes remain focussed on a stationary object when the head moves. If the head moves one way, then a bilateral eye saccade reflexively moves the eyes in the opposite direction, and the image of what was being focussed on remains stable. In EMDR, the head is held still, and both eyes are repeatably saccaded, from focussing to the far left and then to the far right and back, i.e. repeated full saccades of 1 to 4 cycles per second, but only performed when the abnormally formed re-experiencing memory of PTSD type 1, the abnormally formed engram, is consciously recalled and active. As soon as that recall goes, it has to be re-recalled for the next run of saccades: re-recalled and subjected to saccades until it cannot be recalled in that form at all. Simultaneously, the persistent oscillopsia is, step-by-step and in-step with the engram, converted from abnormal-in-form peripheral vision to normal-in-form stable peripheral vision, confirmable on simple visual testing, and the anxiety level subsides step by step. The normal memory of the event is giving **an account** of what had happened and what had been experienced during that moment, no longer giving an abnormal **re-experience** of what had been experienced during that moment.

Successful EMDR most often appears to have a saltatory, a

step-by-step, progression of the processing of the memory contents. It is *as though* some DNA molecule or molecules are being de-methylated, one-by-one or few-by-few, by the repeated EMDR saccades de-tagging the methyl groups from the DNA.

PTSD type 1 can only be diagnosed with confidence after the age of five years or so. A sudden surge of anxiety from a sudden mental shock could occur at any age before five years. We do not yet know, maybe we shall never know, if an epigenetic modification in response to a sudden surge of anxiety or a sudden mental shock can affect any DNA of the brains of *genome-vulnerable children under the age of five years, especially those with the genome for ADHD impairments later in life*: possibly a mental shock giving rise to an autism-spectrum-like disorder together with ADHD impairments life-long.

During the 30 or so years of the exploratory clinical investigation, no person with PTSD type 1 recounted the traumatic event causing their PTSD type 1, having occurred before the age of five years. Many said they had trauma before the age of five years, but no abnormal re-experiencing form of memory of trauma before the age of five years. We are certainly not saying mental trauma, extremes of sudden high anxiety, has no permanent effect on the brains of those below five or six years of age, particularly on those born with the genome for ADHD impairments.

Part Three of Chapter Eight. A plausibly probable neurobiology of PTSD type 2

PTSD type 2 is a generic dimensional disorder, meaning its defining clinical characteristics, other than it following mental trauma, are those of the general class of 'ordinary' anxiety disorders. Top of Form

Its presence depends upon the history of one or more experiences of frightening mentally traumatic events (including 'mental shocks' with sudden surges of high anxiety) followed soon after— minutes, hours, or days, even weeks—by persisting anxiety and anxiety-related symptoms. There are no unique abnormal symptoms suggestive of 'biological brain damage' as in PTSD type 1, hence EMDR treatment has no effect on PTSD type 2. There is no detectable effect of the person's genome on any of the clinical manifestations of PTSD type 2. There is a wide spectrum of severity, i.e. varying dimensions of how severe the anxiety is, how many, how persistent are the anxiety-related symptoms, how many severe experiences of frightening mentally traumatic events (including 'mental shocks' with sudden surges of high anxiety) have been experienced. The anxiety level is *abnormally* high, in that its persisting severity is out of appropriate proportion when it persists long after the danger has passed. PTSD type 2 has no persisting visual symptoms. There may be brief high-anxiety-related irregular oscillopsia, unrelated in form to the persistent peripheral oscillopsia of PTSD type 1. PTSD type 2 can resolve spontaneously over time, but not always does, depending on circumstances (See paragraph below). There is no clearly defined biological marker to confirm the presence or absence of PTSD type 2. Hence, there is no clear clinical marker to confirm treatment or time has finally eliminated PTSD type 2. There is no reason to suppose the sudden development of PTSD type 1 would prevent the simultaneous or later development of PTSD type 2. Both disorders can arise together in response to experiencing the same mentally traumatic event. There is no reason to suppose the surge of anxiety that engendered a PTSD type 1 would always engender a PTSD type 2 and *vice versa*. If PTSD type 1 and PTSD type 2 are present together, and one or the other is cured, there is no reason to suppose the curing of one would affect the other.

PTSD type 2 can be enhanced in severity and can be prolonged indefinitely by the presence of multiple recurring mentally traumatic events and or circumstances. There are situations of continuing dangerous and tormenting existential circumstances (meaning they are subjectively real for that person) and pragmatic circumstances (meaning they are objectively dangerous or tormenting for all people). These continuing situations can prolong PTSD type

2 long after its onset. PTSD type 2 then becomes less of a 'disor-der' *per se*, more a long-continuing and distressing normal anxiety response to continuing dangers and continuing torments, along with losses of relationships and losses of employment. In other words, they develop a Complex PTSD. These existential situations can be virtually impossible-to-do-anything-about, and are all too often accompanied by untreated PTSD type 1. They arise com-monly among the traumatised victims of childhood and or adult abuse, of terrifying and terrible events of long-continued wartime or events encountered over the long term by police, firefighters, and other first responders, and of the personal consequences of natural events of floods, fires, volcanoes, and earthquakes happening at any time anywhere. The accumulating anxiety and mood symptoms from multiple long-term and recurrent mental traumas can eventu-ally disrupt the developing or the developed personality, hence the novel term Complex PTSD for what is, in effect, a post-traumatic stress personality disorder.

CHAPTER NINE

Finding ADHD impairments and PTSD type 1 together more often than expected by chance.

Does having the genome for ADHD impairments increase the likelihood of developing PTSD type 1, making it appear PTSD type 1 could be heritable? The evidentiary clinical findings suggest yes, that this is so — but common sense tells us neither PTSD type 1 nor PTSD type 2 could possibly be heritable, just as a broken leg from a road accident could not be heritable.

The certainty of a clinical diagnosis of PTSD type 1 is now virtually straightforward. The certainty of a clinical diagnosis of ADHD is far from straightforward, it is more nuanced, a diagnosis all too often difficult to pin down. Studies show that about a third of ADHD's heritability is due to a polygenic component comprising many common variants, each having small effects. ADHD impairments are clinically important. ADHD impairments, together with an experience of a sudden mental shock giving rise to PTSD type 1, are extra-important to the person with the ADHD impairments.

What does 'having an ADHD brain' mean?

It means having inherited a varying number of particular genes from one or both parents that produce a brain with an unusual way, not necessarily an abnormal way, of focussing attention. So, some with

ADHD impairments will have very many of these genes, and some will have very few of these genes, and others will have a varying number of these genes in between the extremes. The genes will manifest themselves varyingly, according to their type and number. The ADHD brain with ADHD impairments has an unusually exaggerated tendency to focus attention on particular issues *of interest to that person at a particular time, and simultaneously resist paying attention to all other issues of lesser interest to that person at that time.* It does this regardless of whether, in reality, those issues of lesser interest being ignored are the more important issues to the societal situation at the same particular time. The 'turning off of attention' from uninteresting issues is not a conscious 'turning off', not a practised habit. It is the way the genes of the ADHD brain control the focus of attention automatically. All animals have a greater or lesser differential focussing dependent on perceived interest, for example, the intense focussing on a predator or on a prey where a momentary distraction can seriously determine the outcome of the critical moment of capture. There is no 'deficit' of attention in an ADHD brain, but there is an unusually skewed differential attentiveness compared with the skew of attentiveness of most of the human population, and an unusually skewed differential attentiveness focussing on endless thinking of solutions of unsolved interesting but troublesome issues.

Some people will have so few ADHD genes that in certain times and less demanding environments, there are no noticeable impairments, and they will not warrant the diagnosis of ADHD, but at certain other times and more demanding environments, there are many more noticeable ADHD impairments, and they will warrant the diagnosis of ADHD. 'Medicine is the art of probability'. Geneticists assure us there is no certain genomic test to distinguish those people with 'an ADHD brain but no impairments' from those with 'an ADHD brain and impairments' and those with 'ADHD-like impairments but without an ADHD brain'. As we shall come to: if all human beings could be able to trust themselves with the availability of amphetamine-like medication, then the inevitable difficulties over the optimum management of ADHD impairments in society would be practicable: there is no manageable optimum, so there has to be a compromise. Therapists are expected to do their best, just as police officers are expected to do their best—most people, not all people, obey the rules, and don't 'speed'.

The environment for someone with an ADHD brain will certainly change for the more difficult should they develop PTSD type 1, and on doing so, they will have many more ADHD impairments—a dual diagnosis of ADHD plus PTSD type 1. There will be no doubt about the diagnosis of PTSD type 1 if they are cooperative.

It can easily be seen that having ADHD impairments combined with a low level of intelligence can be extra disadvantageous throughout life, whereas having ADHD impairments combined with a high level of intelligence can be extra advantageous throughout life. There is a natural spectrum of many possible advantages and possible disadvantages in the other genes one inherits and then in the upbringing, one is given; hence a spectrum of the likely good or not so good effect of ADHD impairments has on the development of one's childhood, adolescent and adult character and personality. There is a wide socio-economic spectrum of helpful psychological, psychiatric, medication and educational help that can be given to— if usefully accepted by— those with ADHD brain impairments.

Not surprisingly, people with ADHD impairments of any age are at risk of being stigmatised and or discriminated against. In the late 1960s, the American Psychiatric Association (APA) had been reluctantly obliged to formally designate that having ADHD impairments was to have 'a mental disorder'. This was solely a convenient way to enable the American Food and Drug Administration (the FDA) to legally regulate amphetamine-related medications for the 'medical treatment' of those having ADHD brain impairments. There are many with an ADHD brain who are far from being disordered or impaired—just bright people who are more interesting to be around.

For those with ADHD impairments, any amphetamine-related

substances, in an appropriately low dose for any one person, have a unique non-stimulating effect on their ADHD impairments. Their brain 'chemistry' is slightly different because of their slightly different genes. In higher doses, any amphetamine-related substances have the same stimulating effect as any dose does on those without ADHD genes. The use of amphetamine-related substances is strictly regulated by the American FDA and other countries' drug regulating bodies. The optimum help given to someone with ADHD impairments comes from a strictly controlled dose regimen of an appropriate dexamphetamine-related medication plus supportive psychotherapy. Unfortunately, long-term strict control of such a medication regimen, plus psychotherapy, is rarely practicable: the best achievable is a somewhat, all-too-often messy, compromise, or a complete failure of help, or the non-availability of anyone qualified to help. Psychiatrists and neurologists may try their best to help but all too often have to tolerate being 'blamed by authority' when the clients they are trying to help are seen to break the rules, abuse the use of the medication, or combine the medication with poorly controlled psycho-active substances and become temporary psychotic nuisances to society. Too many psychiatrists and neurologists are driven to preserve their reputations by avoiding individuals with ADHD impairments: "So sorry," says the secretary, "Doctor doesn't see people with ADHD. Do try another psychiatrist, I'm sure you'll find one. Good luck and Goodbye", or they charge so extravagantly that their clients are only the very well established and best behaved.

For a research professor with an ADHD brain and an extra high intelligence, when hyper-concentrating on complex academic problems, and without distractions from elsewhere, taking amphetamines would be disadvantageous: his or her research needs their useful lateral thinking and hyper-concentration of their ADHD brain. But when the professor is called upon to perform the necessary but uninteresting and boringly mundane administrative tasks associated with being a professor and head of department, taking amphetamines becomes advantageous, even a necessity: they must please the administrating Vice Chancellor if they want to keep their job.

For a pupil at school with an ADHD brain, whose schoolwork depends on not hyper-concentrating on other things of interest to them, then taking amphetamines is advantageous, helping them to pay attention to the mundane and boringly uninteresting school curriculum. But when with friends at weekends, their ADHD brain is in no need of amphetamines: hyper-concentrating on novel ideas, creative impulsivity, and sparkling wit, make them the interesting girls and boys they are, thanks to their ADHD brain. Optimally managing the life of anyone with an ADHD brain is far from simple.

When Albert Einstein, the Patron Saint of ADHD, was at Princeton Institute for Advanced Study in the 1950s, there were many helpful people to tidy up his office and to find his bicycle when he'd failed to concentrate on where he'd parked it in the morning. Had Einstein used amphetamines in 1915 to help with his concentration on the boring-and-uninteresting-to-him work in the Bern Patent Office in Switzerland, the Bern Patent Office might have functioned better. But luckily, without amphetamines, he was able to concentrate more on his own complex relativity theory than on any complex patents. Had he used amphetamines, there might have been no relativity theory, albeit a better functioning Patent Office in Bern.

The diagnosis of the recognition of ADHD, trying to be as certain as possible about a person having ADHD, is complex. It involves getting information from them personally and from the people who know them: asking family members, teachers, colleagues at work—and getting information on their coping skills over various times and in various circumstances. Then getting information on family and extended family members likely to have similar genes. Where and when practicable, there can be a controlled trial of taking a 5 mg. tablet of the amphetamine-related medication, Ritalin: taken by a willing and informed person who, at the time, can be relied upon to self-detect and then self-report the mental effects over the next hour or so, and doing so under supervision; those having ADHD will most likely report a welcomed sense of sleepy calm, an un-cluttering of racing thoughts coming within ten minutes of taking the tablet, and the effect lasting for an hour or so; those not having ADHD are likely to have the opposite, an unwelcomed uncomfortable speeding up of thoughts and irritability lasting half an hour or so. This collected clinical evidence related to the person's past and present behaviours and mental experiences can be the useful overall 'test' for the presence or absence of ADHD, a clinical diagnosis of probabilities, a diagnosis 'as good as it can get' at any age. People, as they age, cannot shed their genes like snakes shed their skins as they grow old. A person is born and dies with their genome intact. If one is born with an ADHD brain, one dies with an ADHD brain, a brain tending to become less troublesome as life becomes more predictable and controllable from growing older and hopefully growing wiser.

What is so special about having ADHD and PTSD type 1 together?

There are many reports suggesting, 'PTSD is in part hereditary'. Some reports say, 'as many as thirty percent of PTSD cases are capable of being explained by genetics alone'. But no one can be born with PTSD type 1. No one appears to get PTSD type 1 if they do not have an experience of a sudden mental shock at some stage in their life after the age of five years or so. There are accidental clinical findings from the approximately 30 years or so of clinical investigation, suggesting there is a heritable predisposition, a heritable extra risk factor, for those with the genome for ADHD, to develop PTSD type 1 in response to experiencing a sudden mental shock at some stage in their life after the age of five years or so.

The first problem in assessing evidentiary clinical findings for a relationship between a heritable ADHD and a non-heritable PTSD type 1 comes with the diagnosis of each disorder. People with PTSD type 1 have the simple Visual Test together with recurrent abnormal flashbacks for the certain diagnosis of PTSD type 1. Clinical-near-certainty has to suffice for the diagnosis of having the genome for ADHD. As yet, there is no genomic test for ADHD. If there is no clinical evidence of ADHD impairments, then the diagnosis of ADHD cannot be made. Remembering, 'Medicine is a science of uncertainty and an art of probability'—all diagnoses have to be as good as one can get.

The second problem in assessing evidentiary clinical findings for a relationship between a heritable ADHD and non-heritable PTSD type 1 comes with the availability of statistical data on the northern European population prevalence of each. There is a rough USA estimate of the prevalence of those of all ages with ADHD being of the order of one in ten. At the present time, there can be no data for the prevalence of PTSD type 1 in the northern European population. There is a rough USA estimate of the prevalence of 'PTSD', 'PTSD' as per DSM 5, being of the order of one person in fourteen. For PTSD type 1 specifically, there could be a somewhat higher prevalence or a somewhat lower prevalence in the general northern European population.

The following evidentiary clinical findings are from the later stages of the thirty-year investigation into PTSD type 1: an estimation relating to having PTSD type 1 and having ADHD at the same time. The findings are readily testable by others. The study is a retrospective analysis of the clinical records. Certainly not a statistically sophisticated result, but a seemingly clinically significant result.

A retrospective examination of the clinical files of a sample of a consecutive 100 of the 1 in 14 or so of the general population of any age over 5 years with PTSD type 1 of any severity and had treatment for PTSD type 1 of any severity, 40 of that 100 with confirmed PTSD type 1 were found to have in addition, confirmed ADHD impairments of any severity. The remaining 60 of that 100 with confirmed PTSD type 1, were confirmed not to have ADHD impairments. Having or not having ADHD and PTSD type 1 was confirmed as well as it is possible to confirm them clinically, as described above.

Now for the other way around:

A retrospective examination of the clinical files of a sample of a consecutive 100 individuals of the 1 in 10 of the population of any age with confirmed ADHD impairments and undergoing treatment, revealed that 30 of that 100 were found to have, in addition, confirmed PTSD type 1, of any severity. The remaining 70 of that 100 were tested and found not to have PTSD type 1 by those same clinical criteria. Having or not having ADHD and PTSD type 1 was confirmed as well as it is possible to confirm them clinically, as described above.

These evidentiary clinical findings appear to suggest the following:

If having ADHD and in need of help were independent of having PTSD type 1, then finding the two together would have a probability of the order of 1/140 or so. But, finding PTSD type 1 together with ADHD in those having treatment for ADHD impairments appears to have a probability in the order of 3/10 or so, and finding ADHD with PTSD type 1 in those having treatment of PTSD type 1 appears to have a probability of 4.2/10 or so.

What can these unexpected evidentiary clinical findings imply?

They could infer that those with ADHD impairments and seeking help for those impairments may have, in addition, a 4/10 or so probability of also having PTSD type 1 of any severity as a result of having experienced a mental shock.

They could infer that those found to have PTSD type 1 as a result of having experienced a mental shock of any severity may have, in addition, a 3/10 or so probability of also having ADHD impairments.

They could infer that those people thinking PTSD type 1 might be heritable perhaps should be thinking of an extra probability for developing PTSD type 1 in response to experiencing a mental shock might be heritable.

They could infer that the persistence of ADHD impairments following successful EMDR elimination of PTSD type 1 may complicate post-treatment full recovery.

How can all this be?

Perhaps the onset of PTSD type 1 could engender ADHD impairments in someone with the genome for the susceptibility to ADHD impairments when no impairments had been clinically evident before the onset of PTSD type 1.

Perhaps those with ADHD impairments may have an increased risk of dangerously compulsive or risky behaviours, physically or verbally, and likely to give rise to experiencing many mentally traumatic events and many mental shocks engendering their PTSD type 1.

Perhaps some variant gene combinations can predispose to the development of ADHD impairments, of any severity, in response to difficult life exigencies, and can also predispose to the development of PTSD type 1 of any severity in response to an experience of a mental shock. PTSD type 1 will appear to cluster in those extended families in which those with ADHD appear to cluster. But, it cannot be evidence for any heritability of PTSD type 1.

Troublesome findings. Mental Health workers may simply diagnose 'Anxiety and Depression' based on the clinical features of both when not routinely reasting to exclude ADHD and PTSD type 1 from the overall diagnosis. People with either disorder may not want to know about having the other if they do not already know.

Anyone involved in mental health diagnosis and management should not ignore the possible presence of PTSD type 1 and or ADHD impairments in any client with whom they are in consultation—the former can be detected or ruled out in 30 seconds or so and a suspicion of the latter in four to five minutes or so.

Those with ADHD and or PTSD type 1 should be advised or best decide for themselves to stay away from careers and environments in which mentally traumatic events and sudden mental shocks are more likely to be experienced----soldiering, being a first responder.

PART TWO OF SECTION TWO

The management and treatment of the anxiety
disorders PTSD type 1 and PTSD type 2

CHAPTER TEN

The simple but reliable, sensitive, and specific Visual Test for the presence or absence of PTSD type 1.

The simple test is specific, reliable, and sensitive for the presence or absence of PTSD type 1, and regardless of the presence of other mental or physical disorders: the exceptions being blindness or uncooperativeness. The Visual Test can be performed by anyone on anyone over five or six years old. It takes far longer to read the 'exacting' details of how to accurately perform the simple Visual Test than the 30 seconds needed to perform it. There is always a need to simply ensure against a voluntary or involuntary false positive or false negative test result, as with all reported subjective clinical tests.

A clinician may well shy away from routinely performing The Visual Test when clients make no complaint of visual difficulties or oddities. But clients can be totally unaware of having PTSD type 1 and if asked if they have it, may well say no, when they do have it. During the later years of the clinical investigation mentioned earlier, and clinically since, routinely asking a client in detail about the presence or absence of a recurrent abnormal re-experiencing flashback memory unique to, diagnostic of, PTSD type 1, has proved less effective than routinely performing the Visual Test for accurately detecting the presence or absence of persistent peripheral oscillopsia, which is also unique to and diagnostic of PTSD type 1.

Persistent Peripheral Oscillopsia.

It has been described in detail in Chapter Four above. In brief: the onset (the instant onset or onset delayed for up to ten seconds) of an illusory perception of persistent and consistent rhythmical oscillation, wobbling, of stationary objects seen in a greater-or-lesser portion of the periphery of the visual field. It is apparent when one eye is covered, and the other eye is steadily fixated on a stationary object and held fixated for up to 10 seconds. The illusory perception of oscillations persists for as long as steady fixation (no blinking, not the slightest eye movement) is maintained.

The specific, reliable, and sensitive Visual Test for the presence or absence of PTSD type 1.

An interpreter will be needed for those not understanding the language of the examiner. The test cannot be performed if the person being tested is acutely anxious—there are many transient and chaotic visual abnormalities during a panic attack or near-panic, which is likely to confuse the test result. (See Chapter Two) The test should be delayed until any acute or near panic has passed.

For the sake of this description of The Visual Test, let us suppose the person performing the test, the examiner, answers to being a male (he, him, his), the person being tested answers to being a female (she, her, hers). If possible, a friend or relative of the person being tested will be present and looking on to reassure her. Her age can be as young as 5 or 6 years. She is asked to close one eye; let us say she closes her left eye, and keeps open her right eye. If she has only one normally functioning eye, the test is still valid. If she sees her whole visual field better at one metre with her glasses on, then she should wear them for the test.

The performance of the Visual Test

1.   Throughout the test, she remains seated.

2.   One of her eyes is covered (let us say her left).

3.   She is asked to focus with her right eye on the pupil of the left eye of the examiner, standing in front.

4.   The examiner's left arm is held out rigid and horizontally.

5.   The fingertips of his left hand must just reach the outer periphery of her right visual field—the examiner's distance from her must be adjusted for her to see his fingertips but no further out: this is an essential detail.

6.   During the ten seconds of the test, she is asked not to shift the fixation of her right eye from the examiner's left eye, or blink.

7.   She is asked to pay strict attention to what, if anything, appears to happen to the examiner's left arm, hand, or fingers whilst her right eye remains fixated on his left eye.

8.   After 10 seconds, the examiner lowers his left arm and asks her to demonstrate with her right arm how his left arm, hand and fingers appeared to her at any time during the 10 seconds of keeping her right eye fixated on his left eye.

Figure One.

The Visual Test for Persistent Peripheral Oscillopsia.

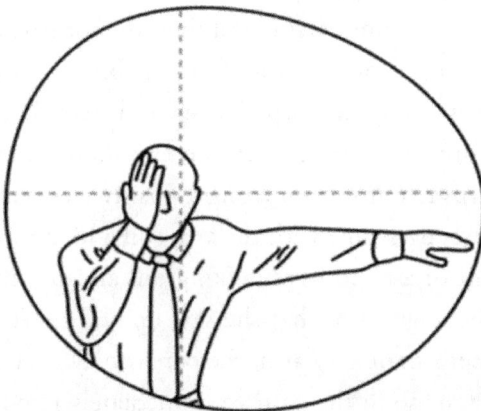

Picture by Silas Tym

How the person performing the test, the examiner, appears to the person being tested during the simple Visual Test. The oval is the outline of the right visual field of the person being tested. The centre of the cross is the visual axis held rigid between the pupil of the left eye of the examiner and the pupil of the right eye of the person being tested. This ensures the person being tested does not momentarily shift fixation unnoticed by the examiner.

The Visual Test gives a positive test result when she (the person being tested) reports: (a) at some time within ten seconds of commencing her steady fixation, some part of the examiner's outstretched left arm, his hand, or just his fingers appeared to swing up and down, or round and round, oscillate, at about two to four up-and-down or round-and-round cycles per second; (b) the oscillations continued uninterruptedly to the end of the ten seconds, or for as long as her right eye remained fixated on his (the examiner's) left eye and his left arm remained extended and stationary.

The Visual Test gives a negative test result when she reports she saw no movement, or she may report she saw only one or two very brief 'jerks up or down' of the examiner's arm during the ten seconds when, in fact, there were no such jerks. Under such circumstances, these are normal visual illusions and of no known clinical significance on the part of anyone who does or does not have PTSD type 1. The jerks do not persist, and they are not part of persistent peripheral oscillopsia or any other form of abnormal oscillopsia.

If there were to be any suspicion she is dissembling over a negative or a positive test result, then the examiner can redo the test and oscillate his left arm, simulating a positive test result, or, have multiple re-tests over time with the arm still and arm moving etc.

If a parent of a child were looking on, and the child demonstrates with her right arm that she saw up and down movements of the examiner's stationary arm, the parent may try (certainly one or two have done so in the past) to immediately remonstrate with the child, "don't be silly, of course, you didn't see that". Parents and others who are present must be asked to remain silent throughout the full test.

Details of the phenomenon, persistent peripheral oscillopsia, experienced during a Positive Test Result, vary from person to person with PTSD type 1 and remain the same for any one person on all subsequent tests over time, over decades, if the PTSD type 1 is not cured (eliminated) or there are further modules of PTSD type 1 from further frightening encounters in the meantime.

For any one person, the oscillations may appear to be there, at each test, from the outset; or they appear at each test only after a few seconds, i.e. there is a constant delay in onset for any one person of from 1 to 7 seconds, e.g., 6 seconds of steady fixation at each session for one person, and 4 seconds of steady fixation any each session for another person.

For any one person, the oscillations, at each test, have a constant extent over the visual field: the extent of apparent movements may be just in the periphery of the visual field, i.e. just the examiner's fingers appearing to oscillate, or more extensive with his hand and fingers appearing to oscillate, or more extensive throughout the visual field with his fingers, hand, and forearm appearing to oscillate, or possibly throughout the whole of the visual field, with the whole examiner and his arm appearing to oscillate.

For any one person, the section of the arm appearing to oscillate may appear to be detached or to be bending as though hinged.

During successful EMDR treatment (see the next Chapter Eleven), as EMDR continues and there is a steady step-by-step degradation of the details of the last remaining module of PTSD type 1, there is a simultaneous steady step-by-step and in-step degradation of all features of the oscillopsia seen on serial visual testing in between the runs of saccades of the final EMDR treatment sessions.

If, at any time, there is even a fragment of an abnormally formed engram remaining evocable, then there will be some minor degree of peripheral oscillopsia remaining.

The Visual Test gives a positive result for PTSD type 1 before successful EMDR treatment and gives a negative result immediately after properly performed successful EMDR has successfully permanently eliminated every module of PTSD type 1: this is the evidentiary clinical finding-b for the effectiveness of EMDR in successfully eliminating PTSD type 1 for that person, regardless of any other mental disorder still-persisting, e.g., PTSD type 2, a psychotic or other mental illness.

Some people with severe PTSD type 1 have oscillopsia of all stationary objects throughout their whole visual field persistently, with no delay in onset and present all day every day, either with their head and eyes held perfectly still or with their head and eyes moving about. Experience shows that EMDR is less likely to be effective in those with such severe persistent peripheral oscillopsia.

CHAPTER ELEVEN

The simple and proper performance of EMDR trial treatment of PTSD type 1.

There are no 'stages' of EMDR treatment. Properly performed EMDR treatment is limited to trial-treating properly diagnosed PTSD type 1. It is not possible to predict with any certainty whether a person with PTSD type 1 can respond successfully to EMDR treatment until properly performed EMDR treatment is tried and persisted for a shortish period of time. For persons of certain genotypes, EMDR is usually a successful treatment for permanently eliminating their PTSD type 1. Persons of certain other genotypes with PTSD type 1 are usually unable to respond successfully to EMDR. The evidentiary clinical evidence strongly infers that PTSD type 1 is caused by an epigenetic insertion and that successful EMDR effects an epigenetic reversal, but we have no idea how or why a person's genes get themselves involved in the biology of EMDR for PTSD type 1.

EMDR has not been proven to successfully treat any other mental or physical disorder. There is good theoretical reason to suppose only EMDR could be expected to cure PTSD type 1 totally and permanently. (See Chapter Eight above.)

It is not necessary for the person with PTSD type 1 to reveal to anyone, the therapist included, what event(s) caused their PTSD type 1 (or PTSD type 2) or reveal the contents of the abnormal recurrent re-experiencing memory flashback(s) or any other memories: the person's privacy is paramount. They can discuss them with anyone if they wish to.

Virtually anyone anywhere can properly diagnose the presence or absence of PTSD type 1 using the Visual Test, and then virtually anyone anywhere can *attempt* to eliminate PTSD type 1 with properly performed EMDR for anyone over 5 or 6 years old with PTSD type 1. Both the Visual Test and EMDR treatment can be performed just behind the battlefield by a paramedic or colleague, or in the living room at home by a parent or friend. EMDR treatment can be as equally effective for children aged 5 to 6 years and older with PTSD type 1 as it can be for adults.

There appear to be genomic factors in some people with PTSD type 1 militating towards a greater severity of their persistent peripheral oscillopsia and towards greater difficulties over their response, if any response at all, to properly-performed EMDR treatment. The evidentiary clinical findings have been that those people with the general genotypes of Northern Europeans with light skin and hair and light-coloured eyes are more likely to have less extensive persistent peripheral oscillopsia and are more likely to (no certainty to) respond to EMDR, than those with the general genotypes of southern Europeans and Iberians with olive skin and dark eyes and dark hair, regardless of their nationality or culture.

Anxiety relief, with conventional medication or other, and always with supportive talking, are part of the overall supportive management of PTSD type 1. For many with PTSD type 1, the intense anxiety, even at the thought of EMDR and having to voluntarily evoke an abnormal flashback during it, is a major reason for some to refuse even to try the treatment. This intense anxiety of voluntarily recalling an abnormal flashback may need to be assuaged by anti-anxiety medication or by some other substance of the person's choice. Perhaps the carefully **controlled use** of cannabidiol **(CBD), or whatever else is preferred and safe, possibly including strictly**

controlled MDMA under the close supervision of an authorised medically qualified person.

A trial of properly performed EMDR aiming to cure correctly diagnosed PTSD type 1.

Let us say the person with PTSD type 1 being treated with EMDR answers to being called a male (him, he, his), and the therapist answers to being called a female (her, she, hers). If possible, a friend or relative of his can be present and looking on, to reassure him. His age can be as young as 5 or 6 years. EMDR treatment is equally effective for those with poor vision or who are blind in one eye. Glasses need not be worn. For those who do not understand the language, an interpreter will be necessary. Blind people with PTSD type 1 have not been seen in this study, but it is reasonable to suppose a trial of simply modified EMDR treatment could be equally effective.

To start, he sits comfortably in a chair. She, the therapist, sits or stands in front, a metre or so away. He is asked to re-evoke one recurrent abnormal re-experiencing flashback memory (perhaps one of several) and then to 'hold' that one flashback—tolerating the re-experiencing of the anxiety and other sensory and physical unpleasant contents of the flashback. This 'holding the flashback' may raise his anxiety to a near-unbearable level, and he will need reassurances that his anxiety will be at its most severe only with the first trial or two of EMDR, and he must do whatever he can to tolerate the discomfort at the beginning of the EMDR treatment. It is at this stage that anxiety-relieving medication, conventional or un-conventional, can be most useful, even necessary.

As soon as the recalled abnormal flashback memory is 'held,' he has a run of repeatedly moving his eyes from side to side, from far left to far right, a run of eye saccades. He does this by following her moving hand with his eyes, keeping his head still, as she repeatedly sweeps her hand in front of him, from far left-to-far-right-to-far-left . . . at one to three sweeps per second.

He is told to stop the run of his eye movements as soon as his abnormal flashback sensation goes, and then she stops her hand-sweeps. This disappearance of the sensation, image or whatever, may have taken a run of just several saccades, i.e. several of her hand-sweeps, or a run of ten or twenty or thirty or more, possibly up to a hundred of her hand-sweeps. If the flashback sensation, image, or whatever will not change in the slightest bit, despite repeated pro-longed runs of saccades, then the EMDR is likely to fail; his genome may render his PTSD type 1 to be EMDR-treatment-resistant.

Assuming the abnormal flashback disappears after a run of saccades, the procedure is repeated several or more times during a treatment session of half an hour or so. He has the same abnormal flashback re-evoked each time, and each run of saccades is contin-ued until the image goes.

If EMDR is being effective, then following every few runs of saccades, he says that he senses the repeatedly re-evoked image (or other sensations if there is no visual image in the flashback) appears to be degrading step-by-step, degrading in its intensity of visual detail, the intensity of sensation, the slightest bit, and he says his anxiety is lessened the slightest bit: the visual detail and colouring of the image is less, the hearing detail is less, his pain is less, the smell has gone . . .

The sessions of runs of eye saccades must continue until no tiny fragment of the abnormal flashback image or sensation can be re-evoked on trying hard to re-evoke a tiny bit of it, and the partic-ular abnormal re-experiencing flashback memory is fully replaced by the same memory in normal non-re-experiencing form. It may have taken as few as one, two, or three runs of eye saccades at the person's first session, or it might have required several sessions, once or twice per week, of repeated runs of eye saccades over weeks or even several months of repeated sessions, before no fragment of his last abnormal flashback image(s) can be re-evoked and it is perma-nently eliminated—replaced by the same memory or memories in normal non-re-experiencing form.

If there are other modules of PTSD type 1, then each module must be fully eliminated by subsequent sessions of runs of saccades.

The full effectiveness of EMDR in permanently eliminating PTSD type 1 can only be verified by a total absence of persistent peripheral oscillopsia on finally repeating the Visual Test.

CHAPTER TWELVE

What treatments are best for PTSD type 1, PTSD type 2 and Personality Disorder Complex PTSD?

Making a diagnosis of PTSD type 1, PTSD type 2 or Complex PTSD, and treating PTSD type 1, PTSD type 2 or Complex PTSD, does not require anyone having to know what specifically caused the PTSD type 1, PTSD type 2 or Complex PTSD for the person, or the specific contents of their recurrent memories of the event or events having caused them. They may want to talk about them, or they may not. Privacy is paramount. What *is* needed for diagnosis and treatment of PTSD type 1, PTSD type 2 and Complex PTSD is ascertaining the exact details of the form of the recurrent memories together with the result of the Visual Test. Anyone with PTSD type 1 may also have PTSD type 2 with or without Complex PTSD—let alone have ADHD, and or a major depressive illness, alcoholism, a prior personality disorder . . . in addition.

A parent can diagnose their five to six years or older child's PTSD type 1 at home and then try treating their child with EMDR. It is possible to self-diagnose PTSD type 1 and possible to try treating oneself with EMDR. For one's own PTSD type 1, perhaps a close friend can teach themselves or be told how to properly perform EMDR and he or she does the EMDR for one's own PTSD type 1.

EMDR is more difficult when there are many different recurrent abnormal flashbacks, a multi-modular PTSD type 1, each module possibly necessitating many sessions of EMDR saccades to totally eliminate. And made much more difficult when the anxiety of each module is severe. Properly performed EMDR treatment for multi-modular PTSD type 1, taking a year or more to complete, is better than suffering PTSD type 1 for the rest of one's life.

The person with PTSD type 1 who does not respond at all to properly performed EMDR requires exposure therapy, together with psychotherapy, possibly anti-anxiety medication or other anti-anxiety substance, and psychosocial intervention: 'good psychotherapists treat the disorder; excellent psychotherapists treat the whole person with the disorder', to parody William Osler's adage.

There are encouraging reports suggesting that strictly controlled cannabinoids, even MDMA, together with Exposure Therapy, may be a breakthrough in the treatment of EMDR-treatment-resistant PTSD type 1 and PTSD type 2. Recent trials are said to have shown MDMA to have some special efficacy in the treatment of a 'PTSD' that has been proven resistant to conventional treatments—presumably to include EMDR treatment-resistant PTSD type 1. Brain imaging studies are said to have shown MDMA reduces activity in the amygdalae nuclei and the hippocampi, which may explain how it helps patients overcome every skerrick of the emotional reliving of traumatic memories.

For the newly arrived patient with severe 'PTSD' the first help is the acknowledgment of their genuine distress. Best not to give reassurances they're now quite safe, no longer anything out there to be worried about—something they are highly likely to know already, and it is not the time for platitudes or paternalism. It may not only be what's 'inside their head' distressing them—physical injuries need to be known about, and as long as they have no concurrent head injury, they may warrant safe conventional pain relief and sedation. Best not to say, ". . . don't worry, it can all be fixed . . ." because there is never any certainty it can all be fixed. And best not to examine too early to see whether it is a PTSD type 1, PTSD type

2 or both—there is no hurry, but it must be done sooner rather than later. (In Chapter Thirteen, Case 2, the woman's PTSD type 1 was diagnosed and permanently cured with EMDR, all within one hour or so of the onset of the PTSD type 1.)

They need to be told that PTSD type 2 may well go away on its own, but not the PTSD type 1. No one wants to be treating a person with normal-in-form, highly distressing memories of PTSD type 2 with EMDR: nothing happens.

What not to do for anyone with any 'PTSD' is to try to talk about it with them when they do not want to be talked to about it, and do not want to talk to anyone about it. A battle-hardened combatant with severe 'PTSD' would likely scoff, angrily saying, ". . . you've no idea what it's like. . . you've no idea what you're talking about . . ." All very understandable. For a combatant, there may be intense bitterness because PTSD type 1 was not the outcome she or he would have expected from their voluntary involvement in deadly combat. Likewise, someone who has been sexually assaulted would likely turn red and say, ". . . thank you, but I'm not going to talk about any of it . . .". A sexually abused person or victim of domestic abuse may well have many different reasons for intense reluctance, if not a refusal, to say what happened. Highly emotive issues evoke high emotions, making people highly emotive. People just want to get rid of their PTSD type 1 and PTSD type 2, a lot more than they want to talk about it. Therapists must make a correct diagnosis, but this does not depend on their knowing what happened, or what the memories are about. Recurrent bad dreams can respond to medication such as Prazosin, an alpha-1 antagonist usually prescribed to treat high blood pressure.

Most PTSD of any severity among non-combatants and non-first responders is found among far-from-wealthy civilians. They are the unemployed young adults, those with ADHD and who drink too much, with limited or no careers; those involved in domestic violence and ousted from home; unhappy unmarried mothers scratching a living—the sexually molested, the sexually abused, and all have many other urgent social and emotional problems.

There is always danger in terms of self-harm or suicide at any stage, at any age, from untreated or un-noticed PTSD type 1, PTSD type 2 or Complex PTSD—all worse when combined with an un-noticed Major Depressive Disorder, unnoticed Schizophrenia, unnoticed frustration with ADHD impairments, un-noticed complex grief, un-noticed drug and alcohol dependence, with un-noticed but endless other social stressors . . . William Osler again, The good physician treats the disease; the great physician treats the patient who has the disease. This is highly applicable to anyone involved in the clinical management of the many problems invariably associated with any post-traumatic stress disorder.

Not everyone who develops a PTSD type 1, PTSD type 2 and Complex PTSD has it recognised by those with whom they work or those who oversee them at work. There are always many members of the police, the firefighters, the ambulance paramedics—all first responders; and the bank tellers and shopkeepers and their assistants—all on the front line, with unrecognised PTSD type 1 and or PTSD type 2 or even Complex PTSD. And not forgetting 'battered wives' who cannot escape the relationship. They all need protection from those who have power over them, those who do not understand or even care what they might be suffering or know they're suffering at all. Colleagues and superiors can all too often be scathing about someone's endless complaining, their changed character and demeanour, their times off work with sick leave, leaving fellow workers short-staffed and overworked in the same dangerous environments. Many are restricted by their proprietorial superiors or their Work Associations from seeking unbiased independent medical/mental help, and are likely to be sent off for assessment by a known-to-be-biased, hired-gun 'expert', a psychologist or psychiatrist well versed in denying that the experience or experiences caused their problem matches the DSM or ICD diagnostic criteria of a 'PTSD', so they cannot possibly have a 'PTSD'.

These are the all-too-often and inevitable injustices meted out to locked-in powerless people of any system. Sooner or later, preferably sooner, they need to be diagnosed: is there PTSD type 1 present, or is there no PTSD type 1 present; do they have PTSD type 2 and Complex PTSD? They need to have the Visual Test explained to them, and have it properly performed, and then re-performed to check—all takes three minutes and costs nothing. There is no reason why any doctor or psychologist or nurse or mate anywhere could not do the simplest of tests, understand the basic PTSD type 1, and do EMDR themselves, performing it properly and then knowing whether it has worked or ensuring someone's PTSD type 1 is taken notice of by someone somewhere. Four percent (at least) of the population is a lot of people with one or other form of 'PTSD'.

There were many men and women, the occasional ex-police-woman seen by this psychiatrist included, who long remain rejected, alienated, abandoned by employers and colleagues alike, left to the dogs of being friendless, pension-less, penniless, homeless, eventually having drug-addicted lives, wishing they were dead but unable to kill themselves, and with severe PTSD type 1 and PTSD type 2 combined, culminating in Complex PTSD, a near-permanent deteriorated personality with features akin to Borderline Personality Disorder or a lot worse. There certainly are some who are quite untreatable without hospitalisation, hospitalisation often refused by the victim and the hospital alike, neither being inclined nor able to afford it anyway.

Some other people with PTSD type 1 of mild severity actually treasure their flashbacks, saying they act as reminders, warnings, to stay away from where the PTSD type 1 had originated, perhaps claiming PTSD type 1 has 'evolutionary protective value'. Many with mild PTSD type 1 and ADHD have neither noticed it until they happen to be asked about it or happen to be tested for persistent peripheral oscillopsia in a routine psychological or psychiatric examination—highly unlikely to happen, alas, in most routine psychological or psychiatric examinations at the present time.

Heart attack, cancer, and all threatening physical illnesses, are endless sources of traumatic stress to the sick person themselves and to those emotionally close. A sudden mental shock from a panic attack or other illness-related frightening moment might arise for either or both the victim and the loved one who is caring for them at any stage. There are many reports of Cancer and PTSD. A study published by the American *Cancer* Society (ACS) estimates twenty-two percent of people with *cancer* have 'symptoms of *PTSD*' six months after their diagnosis. I doubt the ACS knows much about 'PTSD" as yet. Suffering any severe disease can give rise to many non-specific anxiety-related symptoms common to PTSD type 1 and PTSD type 2, without there being anything disordered about their mental distress. Everyone with any form of untreated or untreatable PTSD type 1 will die with it eventually, some from it at their own hand.

Pregnancy and childbirth can be unalloyed rewarding experiences; they can occasionally be very painful, sometimes far too painful, and sometimes distinctly frightening experiences. Giving birth can be followed by Post-Natal Depression; it can be followed by grief; and it can be followed by PTSD type 1 and or PTSD type 2—all in need of recognition and management. Having any form of PTSD does not prevent one from getting pregnant and giving birth. PTSD type 1 is best specifically looked for routinely after a difficult childbirth, and PTSD type 1 is swiftly gotten rid of by EMDR treatment if there, and if possible. The same goes for those women following a miscarriage or an abortion.

Those talking about Mental Health in general rarely advocate deliberately seeking out unrevealed PTSD type 1, PTSD type 2 or Complex PTSD. PTSD type 1 and or PTSD type 2 and ADHD are not infrequently present in those with other disorders, such as Anorexia Nervosa, providing triggers for suicidal ideation. Difficulties in Mental Health Services are not all solved by more and more money—there is always room for more and more awareness and recognition of common multiple mental health disorders, for triple, quadruple diagnoses. Problems tend to add up, self-esteem tends to slither down, and suicidal ideation fluctuates wildly — multiple diagnoses need to be recognised and dealt with serially. Following suicide, a pre-existing ADHD or PTSD of either type does not show up on a physical autopsy and is mostly overlooked in any psychological autopsy if there ever is one. To use the term SLS, standing for 'Shit Life Syndrome' may sound slick and perceptive on the part of some General Practitioners, the doctors plagued by endless patients with endless misery from miserable lives, but hopefully, it is only so graphically used once everything abnormal that can be helped has been excluded. Misery from miserable lives is, sadly, not abnormal.

Grief engendered by the painful death of a loved one, a mixture of to-be-expected anxiety and depressed mood, may have intrusive but normal 'veridical hallucinations'—seeing a 'true picture' of the loved one appearing in a familiar setting, looking just as they were when alive. In addition, the person *may* experience a persistently recurrent abnormal flashing-back memory of some frightening moment around the time of their loved one's painful death. Grief may need more than standard grief counselling. It only takes 30 seconds to perform the simple and hardly obtrusive Visual Test to diagnose or exclude a PTSD type 1 that is permanently complicating and endlessly prolonging the grief if it is ignored.

Treating Complex PTSD means making sure the PTSD type 1 and or PTSD type 2, if present, can or cannot be eliminated by EMDR and or Exposure Therapy, no matter how long ago the traumatic events had occurred. Once again, the therapist does not need to know what happened, why, or when. Providing psychotherapy for the associated 'personality disorder' symptoms caused by the traumas, involves understanding one is dealing with the personality of the disorder, the symptoms, not the personality of the person. The person cannot be blamed for the symptoms when in therapy. The therapist is there to mitigate the effects the symptoms have on the person themselves and on those with whom they routinely

interact. Complex PTSD can be of any severity and of any duration and can co-occur with any other mental or physical disorders,
including, as always. Schizophrenia — there is always 'a mental
health crisis' somewhere in the Western World, if not everywhere.

CHAPTER THIRTEEN

Five short vignettes of clinical management of 'PTSD'

Clinical Case 1.

Corporal Peter's successful elimination of PTSD type 1 by EMDR fifty-five years after the traumatic event in the Korean War. Successfully treated with EMDR at home, first by his wife, then by his next-door farmer's wife.

He first presented at 75, an old-age pensioner who lived 250 miles from my office. He had joined the Army at age 18, in 1950, and had been in the Korean War. He left the Army as a Corporal in December 1953, five months after that war ended and fifty-four years before his consultation with me. Both he and his wife complained that since leaving the Army, he had never been free from anxiousness, had never slept well, had constant nightmares about anything at all, constantly on edge, recurrent headaches, difficulties in concentrating and being always grumpy and jumpy. He was otherwise fit physically despite his age.

On being asked if anything had gone wrong for him in the Korean War, he replied he had not been anywhere near any action and had not been wounded. His wife confirmed he was perfectly fine mentally and physically before joining up and going to Korea, but not at all fine mentally since he returned home. They had sought help on many occasions but were told his "nerves had given out" and the like.

The Visual Test result indicated he had persistent peripheral oscillopsia; he had PTSD type 1. On closer questioning, he spoke of having been involved in a jeep accident. He could only clearly remember a certain moment of the accident but could remember that certain moment very clearly despite the fifty-four years that had passed. The jeep had rolled, and he found himself trapped beneath it, with his mate trapped beneath the front, both fearing at any moment the jeep, poised precariously, would topple over and kill both of them. There was nothing they could do. The next jeep came along ten minutes later, and others started to first lift the front end to release his mate. As they did, he saw the back end of the jeep, slowly at first and then more quickly toppling onto him. He told me, "I felt at that moment terrified it was about to crush me, and that would be it." But the jeep had been held. He, too, was soon released, uninjured. He was back on duty the next day. Such incidents were commonplace at the time, and they were not reported.

He was then eager to talk more. "Just about every day from then till now, I get quick flashes of that dark back end of the jeep coming down on me, like a big black shadow. I keep getting pictures of it coming down, flashing back every day or so. Seeing it, I get the same terrified feeling I had at the very moment I saw it coming down. It's still like the Jeep accident happened just yesterday. My poor wife, I don't know how she's put up with it all these fifty-odd years; we have hardly any social life; I like it when we keep to ourselves . . .." It was quite clear he had PTSD type 1 for the past 54 of his 75 years of life.

There was an immediate trial of EMDR. After half an hour, and with his full cooperation, there was, he said, just the slightest suggestion perhaps the 'picture' was a tiny bit less frightening. A repeat of The Visual Test showed no change—the oscillopsia came after two seconds or so, just as much, and over the outer half of his visual field as before. He was certain there was only one recurring flashback 'picture' of the one 'event'. No, he could not afford the

500-mile round trip to return for more treatment next week—and probably not next month either. His wife was promptly taught to properly perform EMDR, the lesson taking no more than five minutes. It was agreed they would be in touch by telephone. They drove the 250 miles back home. In 1953, when the accident had happened, the name of the disorder was still Traumatic Neurosis, but his was never called even that.

After the fourth week, he answered the phone with, "Yes, there's some definite progress . . . about a third better, I think . . . I can't be sure . . . but there's certainly a bit of a difference in the picture when I get it back . . . it's a bit less scary than before . . . a bit less clear . . . my wife's had to go blueberry picking as she always does at this time of the year, so the neighbour comes in every other day and does the treatment, whatever its name, for half an hour or so . . .". There had been a passing-on of the 'skills' of giving EMDR treatment to the next-door neighbour, a simple 'see one, do one, teach one'. Properly performed EMDR treatment can certainly be 'not difficult' once one knows what PTSD type 1 is.

At eight weeks, his wife had returned and had resumed EMDR. By phone, they both said all had changed. He could not get any bit of the picture back anymore. He felt very much better than ever he could remember. He was sleeping like a baby and having no nightmares. His wife said, ". . . and it's nice to have my husband back after fifty or so years . . .".

On re-attending, seeing him for the second and last time, twelve weeks after his first visit, there was no peripheral oscillopsia on re-performing the simple Visual Test. On questioning, he reported, ". . .yes, of course, I can remember the accident, but it seems vague and a very long time ago now . . . there's no feeling to it . . . I can remember what the picture was, but I can't see it anymore . . . that memory's all fading and it's good to have my life back after all these years . . .you've no idea how I enjoy a night's sleep . . .". Occasionally being in touch by telephone for a year, all remained well.

Clinical Case 2.

Successful elimination of PTSD type 1 with EMDR treatment one hour after the causal event: a woman who did not waste any time before getting help from EMDR.

A middle-aged administrative office worker who happened to work in the building adjacent to my office building attended for a post-treatment check-up. She had been seen with PTSD type 1 six or so months previously and had been successfully treated with EMDR, success confirmed by a positive test result for persistent peripheral oscillopsia before EMDR treatment and a negative test result following treatment. The Visual Test during this follow-up visit confirmed the absence of persistent peripheral oscillopsia. She confirmed that since that last EMDR, she had no abnormal flash-backs as she had experienced before EMDR treatment. She had been back at work and felt she was back to her normal self. She was advised that, being better, she had no need to return.

Surprisingly, she did return—at 9 am the following morning as an emergency, the day after the successful follow-up visit, and in a state of intense agitation. By sheer coincidence, at 8.30 am that morning, she had experienced a moment of instant, sudden and intense fear from an unexpected and out-of-control event in a dys-functional elevator. She had been alone in the elevator. The elevator had suddenly stopped halfway between floors, had suddenly jerked downwards about a metre, and violently, with a terrifying-to-her crashing sound, jolted to a halt. The elevator doors immediately part-opened between the two floors, revealing the dark, bare con-crete walls of the elevator shaft and elevator cables. The elevator alarm went off at the same instant. She had screamed in panic, not daring to move. She was stuck there alone for what seemed ten minutes, panicking and shouting for help but hearing no response. Suddenly, the doors gently closed, the elevator slowly descended to the ground floor, and the doors opened. A security guard was there to help should any help be needed. As she left the elevator, now back on the ground floor, she was still panicking. Within minutes, she asked to be taken to the psychiatrist's office in the adjacent building. She went straight away and sat, panicky and shaky, in the waiting room. She settled somewhat with a cup of coffee from my secretary.

At nine-fifteen, I saw her. The Visual Test that had given a negative test result eighteen hours previously, revealed a return of persistent peripheral oscillopsia, which was the same but more pronounced than it had been six months before. The 'wavy vision' was not chaotic, not that of a near-panic attack. She also had a return of recurrent abnormal flashbacks, this time of the most frightening moment of being stuck in the dysfunctional elevator three-quarters of an hour or so ago. The abnormal flashback was of the part-open elevator doors and the dirty walls of the elevator shaft and elevator cables. She could also re-hear the crash as the elevator had suddenly come to a halt and the screaming alarm. The abnormal flashbacks had been recurring every few minutes since the terrifying event, even recurring whilst in the waiting room drinking her coffee. She was repeatedly re-living the terrifying moment of looking at bare concrete walls and cables and fearing the elevator was about to crash down at any second. There was no other 'picture' flashing back— no other recurring abnormal flashback from that experience in the dysfunctional elevator.

She was treated there and then with EMDR. Her brand-new PTSD type 1 was eliminated there and then within fifteen or so minutes of runs of saccades. Before she left the office, at around 10.30 am, she had no peripheral oscillopsia on visual re-testing. She could now recall her experience in the elevator in a normal fashion, without any re-experiencing extra panic and without re-seeing the picture of what she had seen of the blackened elevator shaft wall through the part open doors of the elevator. She could no longer re-hear the crash. She could remember it all quite clearly. It was now certainly a very unpleasant intrusive memory, but not in any abnormal form. When she left the office, she was still 'shaken up' with

PTSD type 2: she had an only-very-slowly-subsiding PTSD type 2, (a slowly subsiding Acute Stress Reaction in DSM 5 parlance).

She later said, on a follow-up visit, that she had been unable to summon up the courage—unable to overcome the once-bitten, twice-shy fear—to re-enter the same elevator for several weeks. Her 'near-instant' recovery from PTSD type 1, with virtually immediate successful EMDR treatment eliminating it, did not coincide with her recovery from her PTSD type 2, which had arisen at the same time from the same mental shock. On further follow-up, her PTSD type 2 settled slowly over several weeks before she was reusing the same elevator. She was grateful for the weight loss and extra fitness from using the fire escape stairs to get to and from the office for several weeks instead of using the elevator.

Clinical Case 3.

Total failure of EMDR to eliminate multi-modal PTSD type 1. There was precious little anyone could do for her most severe EMDR treatment-resistant PTSD type 1, in effect, a **Complex PTSD** deterioration of demeanour. Perhaps "controlled CBD or even MDMA, plus psychotherapy," will be the answer or lead the way to what will be the routine answer for the management of such a case.

She was a forty-year-old woman, born into a close and religious family from southern Italy. She had her initial mental shock and first module of PTSD type 1 when her first husband died, literally in her arms, during an asthma attack. Her next mental shock, and second module of PTSD type 1, was when she was called to give evidence in the Coroner's Court. Her parents-in-law, in court also, had stood up and publicly blamed her for causing the death of their son by failing to save him. Some weeks later, on returning to work, she suffered a third mental shock and third module of PTSD type 1, when she was verbally sexually abused and screamed at by her supervisor for being too slow. She presented with three modules of PTSD type 1.

She presented with extreme levels of anxiety. Only with great difficulty could she speak of endlessly recurrent abnormal flashbacks of each of the three moments—the blue face of her fighting-for-breath dying husband; the faces of her ex-parents-in-law accusing her in court of failing to save their son's life; her supervisor shouting obscenities at her from across the road.

She had persistent oscillopsia over her whole visual field, with every stationary object seen by her to be oscillating, all day and all night when not asleep. She could not read for more than a moment or two because of it. She could piece together some of what she was looking at on television but without much detail. She could not go out in public. She could not take off her dark glasses. She refused to see her general practitioner about her Type 2 diabetes but did take her medication for it. She could never stop her legs from shaking when in any company. In any 24-hour period, she had, at the most, two hours of continuous sleep, lying on the living room couch. She never went to bed at night. The curtains of the house could never be opened day or night. Oddly, she could occasionally drive her car to see her dying father, at her aged mother's insistence, when her second husband (who had been chosen for her by her family, somewhat reluctantly on his part) could not drive her there.

Despite trying many times, she was totally unable to persist with even the first stage of EMDR because of excruciating-for-her anxiety and her terrifying-to-her flashbacks. Her religious family values prevented her from suicide, but she prayed every night for God to let her die. When seen by other psychiatrists at the behest of the Compensation Company by which her treatment costs were covered, she was deemed to be suffering somewhere between hysteria and deliberate uncooperativeness, with no mention being made of any 'PTSD'. When last seen by me, she was no better than when first seen by me three years earlier. Trying marijuana would have been no more acceptable to her than suicide. She accepted only alprazolam, never changing the dose. Her second husband could not entertain the idea of leaving her but was unable to please her in any way or have a life of his own.

Clinical Case 4.

EMDR successfully eliminating PTSD type 1 in a six-year-old girl, surprising her parents, who could hardly believe what she said and what was done and how effective the treatment was: to them, all very mysterious.

A six-year-old schoolgirl attended with her parents. On questioning the six-year-old in the presence of her parents, she said she had a scare at school about six months ago. She said she had been shouted at by her teacher in the classroom in front of all the other children. She had been very frightened. She had been very nervous ever since—too frightened to go back to school and seeing that teacher again. Her parents told of her behaving with persistent nervousness, poor sleeping, frightening dreaming, and undiminishing fearfulness of going back to school. The six-year-old, on specific questioning, said she had constantly recurring abnormal re-experiencing flashbacks (certainly not her words): 'pictures' of the schoolteacher shouting, and of hearing the teacher's shouting voice.

With her parents present, she there-and-then co-operated fully with the simple Visual Test for persistent peripheral oscillopsia. After ten seconds of staring, and then being asked by me to indicate with her right arm how she saw my left arm, she immediately began to swing her right arm up and down over a forty-degree range at about one to two up-and-down swings per second. Her mother immediately remonstrated, saying to her daughter, "Don't be silly . . . of course it wasn't moving". Her mother was reassured. Her daughter then co-operated fully with EMDR treatment, and according to her report, both the recurrent flashback and the peripheral oscillopsia on re-testing were fully eliminated by one single run of saccades lasting 15 seconds. At follow-up by telephone four weeks later, her parents reported that by the end of two weeks, there had been, remarkably, surprisingly to them, a full return of her pre-PTSD type 1 demeanour, and a return to school with the same teacher— the teacher having been told of their child's likely exaggerated psychological responses to overly gruff verbal discipline in front of the whole class.

The issue of whether the child had exhibited ADHD-like impairments at home or at school was not broached. I thought it was probable, but then it was not the time to open that 'bag of worms'.

Clinical Case 5.

Confusion between PTSD type 1 and PTSD type2–a sceptical and angry woman and her sceptical friend and sceptical lawyer, all wanting results and not interested in any fancy technical information about 'PTSD'.

She was a fifty-year-old highish-level Administrative Assistant. Her work involved driving around the countryside and visiting outlying offices. One Monday morning, she had a very frightening accident: her car was sideswiped by another, which sped off. She had been terrified. Her anxiety level shot up and remained, as she said, "way over the top". She just managed to continue driving and working, but she was 'not herself'. By coincidence, and not necessarily because her anxiety made her inattentive, she had another accident the following Friday afternoon. Her car was hit by another coming illegally through a Stop sign. It was not her fault at all, and there was nothing she could have done to avoid the collision. From the moment of the second accident, she could neither drive nor go to work because of the extremes of her anxiety.

She consulted me three weeks later. She had clearly had PTSD type 1. There was persistent peripheral oscillopsia and two recurrent abnormal flashbacks, one from each of the two accidents. EMDR was terrifying for her. Evoking one flashback tended to bring on the other, with the two flashing in and out. Evoking either caused near screaming, shaking, tears and anger. With great encouragement from her very sceptical best friend, who sat with her through the necessary six initially terrifying, always very uncomfortable sessions of EMDR over three weeks, the abnormal flashbacks of each accident, and her persistent peripheral oscillopsia, were eventually eliminated. The Visual Test was giving a convincingly negative test result, quite different from the convincingly positive test result at the outset of the EMDR treatment.

However, she bitterly complained she was no better at all. She was still riddled with anxiety, could not drive, or even think of going back to work. I was able to tell her, her sceptical colleague, and her soon-to-be sceptical lawyer, at least they would be pleased to hear she no longer had PTSD type 1. The response was the same from all three—her lawyer's contribution was, ". . . don't be ridiculous . . . if she hasn't still got PTSD, what has she got? . . . she wasn't like this before the accidents. . . don't mention anything to her Insurance Company or her workplace that she does not have PTSD anymore. . . she knows she is no better . . . her best friend knows she is no better . . . even I as a lawyer can see she is no better . . .". She undoubtedly no longer had PTSD type 1, but undoubtedly, she still had a fierce PTSD type 2 leftover—the three involved were unable, or unwilling, to comprehend, let alone accept.

She did reluctantly agree her flashbacks were nothing like they were; she could no longer 'see' the bright blue flash of the car that had sideswiped her, or the shattered windscreen she suddenly saw at the moment of the second accident. But every time she recalled the accidents, she still had a near panic attack. Her anxiety was such that she could not return to work, and she could not even get into her car, let alone drive it. She was angry, and her friend was angry. ". . . your EMDR treatment or whatever it's called doesn't work . . . anyone can see that . . . she should have seen a psychologist from the start, not you . . .", said the friend. The EMDR had been almost as distressing for her, her friend, to watch as distressing for her, the victim, to bear. By strict DSM 5 criteria, she was still suffering from PTSD, and

EMDR had not worked. The only difference, now, was the absence of the obscure visual abnormality, persistent peripheral oscillopsia, which had worried her not at all, and the obscure memory abnormality, the recurrent abnormal flashback, now replaced by intrusive distressing memories of the same two traumatic incidents.

For her PTSD type 2 she had several months of Cognitive Behavioural Psychotherapy, CBT (mostly exposure therapy) from a neuropsychologist. She made a full recovery from her PTSD type 2 and returned to work and to driving. Distressing memories of the accidents, the anxiety, the EMDR, the CBT, the period off work and all the distress of bitter arguments with the Insurance Company over her entitlements, all somewhat intrusive distressing memories, were still somewhat distressing to her when they were recalled.

There would have been little or no recovery with CBT had there been no prior elimination of the PTSD type 1 with the EMDR treatment, but she, her friend and her lawyer were still convinced the EMDR had been painful and unnecessary.

CHAPTER FOURTEEN

Anorexia Nervosa being mixed up with ADHD, with PTSD type 1 and with PTSD type 2.

Anorexia Nervosa, AN, is a complicated, occasionally fatal mental disorder. There has been, until now, no clinical or other evidence for anything physical—no genomic, immunologic, neurologic, or infective explanation to account for the onset of AN. But as with PTSD type 1, there 'appear' to be genetic factors in AN:

"Knowledge of genetic influences on liability to eating disorders has grown rapidly over the past three decades. Indeed, numerous family, twin, and genetic studies have indicated genetic effects contribute to the variance in liability to eating disorders including anorexia nervosa*."

> *Thornton LM et al. The Heritability of Eating Disorders Methods and Current Findings, pp141-156, in Behavioural Neurobiology of Eating Disorders, Eds. Roger A.H. Adan and Walter H. Kaye. Current Topics in Behavioural Neurosciences, 2011 series.*

Not so fast! At present, AN must be regarded as a "psychological disorder" and requires "brain reprogramming" in the form of family psychotherapy. Clinically, it is not infrequently complicated by associated ADHD, and possibly PTSD type 1, two disorders easily missed if not looked for when trying to cope with someone with something as complicated as AN. Finding a 'cause' of AN is

178 Dr Robert Tym

a challenge to anyone's intuition, their conceptual grasp of things: one is left having to fall back on the person's subconscious mind for an explanation of its 'cause'. Its clinical manifestations are all too obvious: the person voluntarily consumes too little nourishment, is too thin, and is getting dangerously thinner.

The subconscious is that part of the mind 'that notices and remembers information when one is not trying to, and subsequently influences behaviour without one's conscious realisation'. Finding a possible subconscious explanation, a cause, for a mental disorder characterised by inexplicable dangerous behaviour, an explanation to help make a reasoned guess at likely effective treatment, always requires one's intuition, one's informed speculation.

There is the undeniable fact: some highly intelligent female teenagers (not all that uncommonly male teenagers or young adults) develop intense anxiety after they have eaten. Avoiding the intense anxiety following eating means avoiding eating: no one has an appetite for intense anxiety. Undereating leads to dangerous under-nourishment and can eventually lead to death from complications of starvation. No one knows of any physiological mechanism to explain why eating safe and nourishing food can give rise to intense anxiety. The teenager has no idea why eating makes her anxious. She is often forced to consciously rationalise and make up excuses to satisfy both herself and others, others who are forever asking why she has anxiety when she eats. "I'm too fat" is a rational-sounding excuse for everyone. Both not eating, and believing her made-up excuse, relieve her anxiety—she is unconsciously and consciously unlikely to voluntarily do the things that make her anxious: her delusional beliefs are reinforced by being her safeguards from anxiety. Looking at her weight loss tells everyone else her rationalization is irrational; she must be delusional. A delusion is "an idiosyncratic, strongly held belief despite being contradicted by reality". Applying logic to the situation, and trying to reason with her gets nowhere; coercing her to eat more gets nowhere; threats of punishment for not eating get nowhere; rhetoric gets nowhere; antipsychotic medication gets nowhere other than assuaging somewhat her anxiety. A normal brain cannot always remain rational when a belief in a particular irrationality can be so effective in assuaging anxiety. It never occurs to anyone in the family that there is any family problem: "We're a happy, close, and loving family, aren't we, love?" "Yes, Dad, whatever you say."

The condition was described in detail by Queen Victoria's personal physician, Sir William Gull, in 1873. Females depicted in magazines at the time were far from unusually thin. The French called it *De l'Anorxie Hysterique*, the hysteria word again meaning, 'it does not have a physical cause'. To rationalise a person's AN, one has no option other than to talk to a lot of people with AN, to collect observations, to collect thoughts—speculating and learning and at the same time preventing them from dying of starvation.

Informed therapists talk with her about her family relationships. Family relationships are all 'in the eye of each beholder'; and different in the conscious and the subconscious mind of each member of the family. What is provable, what is real, what is false, are not the issues. The therapist has to be speculative: try to detect some logical-under-the-circumstances, likely-to-be-effective explanation, upon which to base an effective 'treatment' strategy, one necessarily unrevealed to the person herself who most probably is not consciously asking for any 'treatment'.

The most useful speculation: a pernicious situation appears to arise if an intelligent teenager consciously convinces herself over time that her father or stepfather or adoptive father, whoever is the most important protective person in her life at the time, the head of her hierarchy, is beginning to favour one or more of her siblings over her, or perhaps favouring some other rival. Rightly or wrongly, she perceives herself as being gently supplanted in the family hierarchy—edged out of favour, and soon to be rejected from 'the nest', dangerously abandoned. Especially vulnerable if she is a twin, or is adopted, or is 'letting the family down', perhaps by unrecognised ADHD impairments: ". . . she just doesn't listen, she's all over the place, she's just a disappointment to the family . . .". In a quite natural response to her perception, she is losing the affection of her father, being a nuisance to him, believing all the more that her father increasingly prefers others to her, and she is in danger of being rejected by him: she is consciously or subconsciously jealous of her rivals. But the 'J' word cannot be consciously acknowledged. Animals kill and get killed over the 'J' word, but polite and intelligent young ladies do not kill, even consciously challenge, their rivals, but they do feel anxious and depressed in mood, helpless and threatened and they don't know what to do.

At this stage, the subconscious mind takes over. The subconscious devises various plans to regain the attention of her father. If she is intelligent, then the likelihood is her subconscious mind is intelligent too. She could self-harm by cutting her arms or thighs and the subconscious would arrange for the cutting to be painless. She could painlessly take an overdose of something. More subtly, the ingenious subconscious could arrange for her to be painlessly underfed and wasting away. One way or another, to avoid the danger of being rejected, she needs to attract extra attention and be extra cared for without asking for extra attention or extra care. Risk-taking behaviours—any one of which can have a fatal outcome—indicate the ruthlessness of an ingenious subconscious mind and the seriousness of the situation in the unconscious mind of the person. Such complex self-harm problems are usually subsumed under the name 'mental health problems. The person needs some special attention but is unable to articulate the facts. All too often, one hears a derogatory ". . . she's (or he's) just seeking attention . . .". To maintain their 'mental health' they certainly need to seek and get attention — but exactly the right sort of attention.

If her father merely tries to cajole her to eat, or worse, gives permission for her to be force-fed to keep her alive, but does this without demonstrating a change away from showing affection for her 'rivals', he merely makes things worse. She presumes she is being seen as a mere nuisance to him. What she needs is conscious evidence, enough evidence to convince her and her subconscious that her father does not prefer others to her; he does accept her as more than an equal in *worth* to any other. Too often, the father truly thinks she is a nuisance for simply refusing to eat for apparently no reason. There can be an impasse: will the father change sides or not? Will he convincingly come over to her side, or will she have to continue self-starving, regardless of the risk of her death?

Here, then, is the therapists' family therapy solution: to gently manoeuvre both a conscious and subconscious reconciliation between a cooperative and understanding father and his previously feeling-rejected starving daughter. Sadly, not every such solution works in time to stop the outcome from becoming a fatal under-nourishment.

The ballet dancer's story: Anorexia Nervosa together with ADHD and PTSD type 1.

A very thin but very intelligent young woman, a year previously a budding principal ballerina in a New York ballet company, could hardly bear to eat because it made her too anxious. She was attending an Eating Disorders Day Clinic. When I first arrived to work there, and first met her, she was still wanting help despite endless group psychotherapy sessions in the very strict clinic. On my first examination of this bright young woman, she had marked persistent peripheral oscillopsia. Being asked, she volunteered, and had no hesitation in relating two very distressing recurrent abnormal flashbacks from having been savagely raped in her New York apartment eighteen months previously. The Eating Disorder psychologists had tried to talk to her about the trauma and the problem of the flashbacks, not mentioning "PTSD", but had concentrated more on the need for her to eat, which she knew quite well was also a problem. She was making little, if any, progress.

Following the sexual assault eighteen months ago, she could not cope with remaining in ballet. Being on stage, any glimpse at the audience sitting in the dark of the auditorium triggered endless abnormal flashbacks: she never knew if 'he', her rapist, was out there watching. She had eventually left New York and returned to the UK and to home, or rather just to her mother's home — her father, with whom she was once very close, now lived elsewhere with another woman. She could no longer talk with either parent, certainly not about any rape to her father or about her anxiety with eating. Both parents had always disapproved of her previous lifestyle in New York. Prior to that, their disapproval had been for doing so badly at her expensive private school despite being highly intelligent, then for abandoning learning altogether and 'going on the stage', taking to dancing. In their view, she had gotten what she deserved for going off to New York alone, against their advice, and now, she had to return home unable to cope, as they had predicted. Her father scathingly saying, "…she is deliberately starving herself, wanting to get thin enough to go back to dancing…"

In one abnormal flashback, she could 're-see' the blue duvet on her bed where the rape was happening, and 're-feel' the dreadful pain of what was happening. On the other, from an equally terrifying moment during the rape, she could 're-see' the blowing curtain of her apartment and 're-smell' the awful body odour and awful breath of the rapist.

It was equally evident, on listening to her, that throughout her younger years, she had marked ADHD-type impairments, which had been the main reason for not being able to cope academically despite her intelligence, and eventually 'going on the stage', becoming creatively independent and looking after herself. Her ADHD impairments soon faded when she took to dancing, now enhancing her intense concentration on highly intelligent dance creativity, boosting her self-esteem and self-confidence.

But ADHD impairments, endless difficulties in concentrating, and endless chattering thoughts had all returned since the sexual assault and its PTSD type 1 aftermath of anxiety and abnormal re-experiencing flashback memories. She could not sustain her independence as before. She had returned to live close to her mother's house and could just be persuaded to accept the Day Clinic's somewhat ineffective talking therapy and the Day Clinic's extra-anxiety-provoking mandatory three meals a day.

She eagerly cooperated with EMDR and was delighted to have the abnormal flashbacks eliminated in four sessions. Also, she was now taking 10 mgs of Ritalin twice a day for her ADHD. Her anxiety level dropped. She found it far less anxiety-provoking when faced with the mandatory meals that had to be seen to be eaten before 'being allowed' to go back to her apartment each night. She began to socialise in the evenings with others from the clinic and managed to start putting back her lost weight. There was no facility for family therapy. But once again, she had become an 'independent equal adult', and no longer needed or wanted any 'loving acceptance' from either parent. Once she returned to New York and to all her ballet friends, she would have her own safe and secure nest, and find it easier to have a good relationship with her parents when far apart from them. And little or no further problem with eating.

The psychologists of the Day Clinic were extra-sceptical about an amphetamine, a well-known appetite suppressant used by the over-weight, now being used in the treatment of a starving, skinny anorexic. Nonetheless, the psychologists were pleased to see one of their favourite clients getting better, assuming it was the clinic's group therapies and the clinic's enticing meals, kicking-in at last. At that time, the EMDR and the 'PTSD' were thought irrelevant, aspects in which only I, the eccentric visiting psychiatrist on sabbatical from Australia, was interested.

Another teenager's story. Anorexia Nervosa plus ADHD; now, plus PTSD type 1.

This highly intelligent sixteen-year-old schoolgirl was referred to me at her mother's request. From an early age, her daughter had been so plagued with such high anxiety when at school that she was eventually unable to go at all. She had home-schooling from her mother. Unnoticed ADHD impairments had led to disappointing her teachers, her parents, particularly her father, and disappointing herself with repeated school failures. She had lived with endless anxiety-provoking criticism from teachers and parents, particularly from her father. Her 'brilliant' older brother excelled in everything at school, cricket included, and was her father's truest friend. Her mother kept her very close. Her father had now left 'home' to live close by with a new female partner.

The onset of Anorexia Nervosa had been obvious to her mother a year previously. In desperation after months of her daughter's intransigence over under-eating, her mother had called for help from the local Mental Health Team. On a home visit by the team, the young fifteen-year-old was deemed to be dangerously thin. Her mother was accused of 'failing to provide due care and protection'. The teenager was declared 'in need of care and protection, needing immediate admission to hospital'. The teenager thought it outrageous and refused to go to hospital but did so when a policeman called at the house to ensure she did. She was detained in hospital against her and her mother's wishes, all sanctioned under the local Mental Health Act.

Despite endless cajoling, she refused to eat in the hospital. This 'desperate situation' of severe undernourishment soon required 'desperate measures': she was duly force-fed. Three nurses, one a male, joined forces to hold her down and force a feeding tube through her nose down into her stomach. She fought, and they fought back. The mental and physical pain of it all made her panic—a mental shock as the tube went down into her trachea to her lungs before being withdrawn and moved down her oesophagus into her stomach. Sadly, this forced feeding for life-endangering Anorexia Nervosa triggered a PTSD type 1 on top of her AN and ADHD. But having been force-fed by a stomach tube, she was safely alive. Over a few weeks, now extra-distressed by her PTSD type 1, and repeatedly being frightened by her abnormal flashback sensations of being force-fed, she eventually succumbed to emotional coercion, slowly eating enough over time to gain enough weight to be allowed home.

I was asked to see her for the first time a month or so after her discharge home from the hospital. There was no hiding her ADHD impairments or her PTSD type 1. The Visual Test showed persistent peripheral oscillopsia. She had recurrent abnormal flashbacks of seeing the face of the male nurse as he grabbed her face with one hand and determinedly forced the tube through her nose with the other.

She soon understood all about PTSD type 1, and soon agreed to have EMDR. Despite every effort over several weeks and with her full cooperation, EMDR had no effect at all. She is a very pale-skinned Caucasian girl, but with very dark brown, almost black irises, and dark brown, almost black hair—both features beautiful to see, but sadly indicating a phenotype making EMDR likely to be difficult if not totally ineffective for PTSD type 1 treatment.

The persisting high anxiety of her PTSD type 1 will be constantly inimical to her mental and physical health and social well-being. She politely declined family therapy with any member of the family but was willing to talk about them. Soon, she was consciously accepting her father's passive rejection. Whenever she visited her father, there were always some women's clothes neatly folded in his bedroom. Her father could never find much to say to her anyway, finding it easier to spend time with his brilliant son, her older brother.

Her father, for certain, has ADHD-related impairments, and soon enjoyed having one or more of his daughter's Ritalin tablets to calm him down, and help him sleep. He had never heard of ADHD until his daughter came home one day with a prescription for Ritalin. With equal certainty, her brilliant brother does not have ADHD.

Were anyone un-subtle enough to ask the bright but now angry young woman, she would certainly deny ever having been jealous of anyone, only angry with the hospital for force-feeding her and with her parents for letting them—though they had had no choice.

Perhaps a never-thought-of-before cause and cure for Anorexia Nervosa is just around the corner. Perhaps a readily available full cure for EMDR-resistant PTSD type 1 is also just around the corner. She now lives in a different country, rarely in contact with her parents. Hopefully, someone will somehow treat her with cannabinoids and exposure therapy. Those involved with Genome Wide Association Studies will hopefully not ignore the problems of those with PTSD type 1 who, mysteriously, cannot respond to EMDR.

ADDENDUM

What is depression, and what are depressive illnesses? What is ECT? Where does "PTSD" fit into Mental Illnesses?

At one time, I was spending a day per week consulting in a nearby small country town. A 70-year-old man of local note, wealth and good standing, was referred to me by his General Practitioner. He arrived together with his wife and son. The story was that two nights previously, he had left the house sometime after midnight without anyone knowing. By lucky chance, he had been spotted at about one o'clock in the morning by a young woman walking home from a party and crossing the bridge of the small country town's sizable river. To the young woman's amazement, she had seen this elderly man wading about in the river below. The water was almost up to his armpits. He had taken no notice of her shouting. The young woman called the police. One way or another, and thanks to the quick actions of the police and the considerable bravery of the young woman who had waded into the icy cold water before the police arrived, he was brought to the shore. He had feebly resisted being brought to the shore—feebly because he was thin, soaked to the skin, and he was all but frozen, certainly hypothermic.

His wife was soon by her husband's hospital bedside. He was warmed up overnight and taken home the next morning on the assurance he would be seeing the visiting psychiatrist, me, within two days. In the meantime, he would not be let out of someone's sight. All doors of the house would be deadlocked. No one wanted him admitted to the nearest Psychiatric Hospital, which was several hours' drive away.

Mr Mill, not his real name, had made it clear he was so depressed, so riddled with guilt, he had wanted to die. He slowly explained how he had been a wealthy man in the past but was now bankrupt—all had been lost and all by his own stupidity. He said there was nothing more to it. His wife said that only her husband knew the financial details and Mr Mill himself would not elaborate any further. When asked further, he stared into space, his face and body virtually immobile, with no eye contact and saying nothing. He was certainly in a very depressed mood.

Both his wife and his son said they knew he was in considerable financial trouble. He had hinted many times over the past two to three months he'd be better off dead. He'd occasionally talked about how good it would be 'to end it all' but promised he would 'never do it'. He had been sitting around all day, day after day, virtually motionless in a chair, ruminating. He had been eating very little, sleeping very little, talking very little. When he did say anything, it was about his being unworthy and unforgivably guilty for having brought shame and bankruptcy on the household and family by so foolishly mismanaging the family's fortune. He had said many times, "…who wouldn't rather die in peace at my age than have the shame of facing the bankruptcy court… I know I'll have to sooner or later…"

His wife was depressed in mood, certainly. She was unsure as to how they would cope. She had been quietly planning to put their large house on the market. His son was curious as to how this hitherto financially smart father had made such mistakes. His wife felt her husband would certainly be doing something about it if there were some things that could be done about it. No one was surprised he was deeply depressed about it all. Everyone felt very sorry for him and said so. There had been a couple of months with virtually nothing coming through the post to cheer him up. He was getting steadily more depressed, thinner, at times confused, inattentive and always uncharacteristically uncommunicative. No one thought for a moment he would try to kill himself. If he had said he was going bankrupt, then there was no gainsaying it. His financial shenanigans had always been secretive but always highly successful until now.

I asked if he had been in touch with his bank manager recently, or whether she, his wife, had. She said she had been told quite firmly by her husband that since the bank manager was a close family friend, she should not contact him. Her husband had said it was too late for the bank manager to do anything anyway, and it would be all too embarrassing. His wife had never been allowed to interfere before and saw no reason to interfere now. He always knew what he was doing.

I eventually persuaded his wife and son, and there and then, that there was no alternative other than to ring the bank manager. Sooner or later, the bank manager would hear, if he had not already heard, the story: the local weekly newspaper, due out in two days, had an editor rarely backward in coming forward with a good story of a brave young woman rescuing a well-known old man from the middle of the icy cold river in the middle of the night.

I rang the bank manager. I explained the situation and the quandary. The bank manager was alarmed. He had no hesitation in breaking confidentiality. I passed the phone to Mrs Mill. The bank manager reassured Mr Mill's wife of an untouched several million dollars and no debts. There had been no financial interactions for the past three months. Dividends were accumulating as expected. The bank manager had assumed all was well. He had seen no reason to interfere with a phone call.

Mr Mill, on hearing the news, assured his wife the bank manager was wrong; the bank manager didn't know or didn't understand. The bank manager had been so alarmed he had left the bank there and then, came to my office and produced a copy of the bank account. Mrs Mill and her son were amazed, grateful and confused. Mr Mill was adamant he was right, and that the bank manager was wrong.

The appropriate psychiatric explanation was given. His wife and son were now convinced Mr Mill was mentally ill, and delusionally so. Not surprisingly, Mr Mill said he wasn't mentally ill. Despite Mr Mill's stated conviction that he wasn't in any way mentally ill, he did agree at the same time to accept medication. Mr Mill said he was taking the medication for no reason other than it would enable him to sleep better, worry less and put back the weight he had been losing. He had not enjoyed his evening in the cold waters of the river. He would certainly be returning home from my office, not going to the hospital. His wife, son and daughter-in-law swore he would never be out of their sight. Doors and windows were to remain deadlocked. Mr Mill was to have no access to a key. Mr Mill's son was to sleep at the house for the next two or three weeks. I emphasised the danger of suicide would not be over for several weeks. The danger of suicide would be increased somewhat over the time that Mr Mill was becoming more energetic as the medication took its initial effect. The medication was a combination of an antidepressant—not effective on its own—and an anti-psychotic. I warned that medication was not always sufficient. ECT may be necessary in view of Mr Mill's age and the severity of the delusional illness. Mr Mill, paradoxically, half knowing and half not knowing the reality of the situation, accepted the full dose of antidepressant and antipsychotic medication. The local general practitioner was now fully aware of the situation and fully attentive.

Over six to eight weeks, he made a slow but full recovery from his psychotic mental illness of depressed mood. After the first four weeks of his medication treatment, he began to say that for the life of him, he couldn't understand why he ever thought he was bankrupt or why he had never bothered to check with the bank. All he knew was he had been very depressed and had assumed, indeed believed, there was, must be, something to be very depressed about.

He was now slowly regaining his normal cognitive functioning, no longer muddle-headed, no longer forgetful, no longer inattentive, no longer irritable—and no longer delusional, his beliefs about the health of his finances now in tune with a normal mental state, a neutral mood. He was moving about normally. His face was having varying expressions. His eyes were looking around and making eye contact. He was walking every day with his wife, regaining weight, sleeping well, and planning a not-inexpensive ocean cruise with his wife. His friends thought it all very odd.

He was no longer having an abnormal, inappropriate and unshakeable mood of depression due to switched-on rogue genes, and no longer had a mood-matching belief in a financial catastrophe to provide an unshakeable psychotic explanation for his unshakeable psychotic mood. Medication had corrected the malfunctioning genes. Rigidly held beliefs must be mood congruent, as in Anorexia Nervosa in the last Chapter. Cognitive dissonance is when there is conflict between two beliefs, both of which cannot be true.

If he ever did subsequently go bankrupt—highly unlikely for him—then he would become very depressed in mood again, and rightly so. Anti-depressants and anti-psychotics would not help his mood then, only money, to cure his real bankruptcy—with enough money, there would be nothing to be depressed about.

Had his switched-on rogue genes malfunctioned the other way, and he had had a Bipolar Illness, he may well have developed an abnormal, inappropriate and unshakeable mood of elation—a psychotic mental illness of manic happiness. There would have been an abnormal, unshakeable psychotic belief, perhaps, of having twenty million dollars in the bank instead of just several. This abnormal, inappropriate and unshakeable psychotic belief of untold wealth would match his abnormal, inappropriate and unshakeable psychotic mood of elation. Were he to start spending the money he believed he must have but didn't have, then he certainly would become bankrupt very quickly. Once medication, more likely ECT, had corrected those malfunctioning genes of manic mood, and he was back with normal brain functioning and no inappropriate manic mood, he would be very and quite appropriately depressed in mood on realising his beliefs in untold wealth had been psychotic and he was now well and truly bankrupt. He would need money and not antidepressant and antipsychotic medication to get rid of his 'normal' depressed mood from finding himself well and truly penniless as a result of a dangerous mental illness-triggered abnormal belief of untold affluence.

Should his rogue genes have malfunctioned in such a way he developed an abnormal, inappropriate and unshakeable emotion of anxiety leading to fear, he may well have developed inappropriate and unshakeable psychotic beliefs congruent with his being persecuted, in some form of danger. Such misperceived dangers may have been a delusional belief of others' conspiracies against him or even of his wife's infidelity. He would have developed a delusional disorder, with abnormal, unshakeable beliefs of persecution and or behaviours consistent with misconceived jealousy. Unfortunately, there is no medication or other curative treatment as yet for Mental Illnesses based on malfunctioning genes giving rise to inappropriate anxiety and their congruent psychotic beliefs—the Psychotic Persecutory Disorders.

The situation for Mrs Mill over Mr Mill's psychotic mental Illness of depressed mood had almost been a 'folie a deux', even a 'folie a famille' if his son and daughter-in-law were to have been included in an unshakable delusional belief of his bankruptcy. This was a 19th century conceptualization by French psychiatrists of 'a shared psychosis', somewhat grandiosely known as the Lasegue-Fairet Syndrome: two or more people equally appearing 'psychotic', in that the mentally healthy ones had acquired the same unshakable false beliefs by accepting and believing the delusional beliefs of their emotionally close psychotic family member. In the case of 'Mrs Mill and her children', they appeared to be equally convinced of his bankruptcy. But such a label would be somewhat of a melodramatic conceptualization. Neither his wife nor his offspring were psychotic;

they were merely misinformed and misled, with little reason ever to doubt the word of the head of the household. None had any ready means of checking, and none had any reason to suspect the honourable man was mentally ill or to entertain an alternative of his actually 'lying' about some clandestine arrangement with some other person who would be getting the family's inheritance secretly.

Mr Mill had been spared ECT. Had he not responded to anti-psychotic antidepressant medication after six weeks, he and his family would have had to be persuaded to agree to ECT. If he had not agreed to have ECT voluntarily, it would have been necessary to invoke The Mental Health Act. He would have been admitted to a psychiatric hospital and against his and his family's will if necessary. He would have had ECT administered. Desperate situations require desperate remedies. ECT would be given against his and his family's wishes if necessary—but only after his involuntary detention in hospital and the ECT had both been sanctioned by the local Magistrate and a second psychiatrist's opinion. Had medication failed and ECT have been avoided by Mr Mill's family employing a smart barrister to successfully contest the magistrate's sanctioning of it, then Mr Mill's life would have been in serious danger sooner rather than later from serious self-harm and or malnutrition.

A final note on ECT.

The aim of ECT is to produce a 'strictly controlled' epileptic fit, a seizure. Seizures have an extraordinary curative effect on some otherwise incurable Mental Illnesses for reasons presently unknowable. For hundreds of years, the 'earliest psychiatrists' had been watching patients with devastating, serious, and many-years-long-standing mental illnesses, inexplicably recover spontaneously, rapidly, and completely, following a coincidental series of major epileptic seizures—the cause of the seizures being unrelated to the mental illnesses themselves. In the year 1500, Paracelsus was giving camphor by mouth to produce seizures in an attempt to emulate the natural occurrences of epileptic seizures in desperately, otherwise incurably mentally ill patients. In 1934, an Italian psychiatrist, Ugo Cerletti, started giving electric shocks to the scalp to produce seizures in mentally ill patients. Seizures aren't easy to produce, safely or pleasantly.

Today, in 2024, necessary ECT is sophisticated and safe. Today, psychiatrists trust ECT. Patients need to trust the psychiatrist and anaesthetist who is giving the ECT. ECT is performed in the hospital. The patient is admitted for a day. The patient is briefly fully anaesthetised and paralysed—the latter to ensure there is no muscle jerking during the 15 seconds of the seizure. The generalised seizure is confirmed and monitored by a scalp electro-encephalogram (EEG). There is either just one ECT electrode held to the right side of the head, or one held to each side of the head.

The voltage varies from 224 to 450, enough to maintain a steady current of 0.9 amps. The energy per second applied to the skull is 85.05 Joules, a power output of 85.05 Watts, (which would be enough power to keep a large light bulb glowing brightly for more than five seconds—an otherwise irrelevant fact to hopefully shed enough light on the exactitude of the ECT's electrical machinations and dispel any mystique). The wattage (the amount of electric power) and the seizure combined, change the brain's metabolism a little, not surprisingly, but not necessarily permanently. The patient wakes up within minutes and, within an hour or two, goes home.

The post-ECT EEG can remain mildly abnormal for several months following a course of twelve or so ECT given over a three-week period, but not indicate any obvious persisting clinical abnormality of memory or of anything else. Recovery from any side effects of ECT, like recovery from traumatic brain damage or an appendectomy for appendicitis, is quicker for the young than for the old. In the case of the brain, there is a degree of neuroplasticity, i.e. the brain's ability to restore some, if not all, lost function after damage.

Memory for events before the ECT may be transiently affected—it is impossible to quantify; it is of some initial annoyance to the patient but is of little long-term significance, as most memory returns. There is no clear evidence of permanent brain damage from ECT—which doesn't mean there is no small degree of permanent brain damage from ECT. Some small degree of permanent brain damage from ECT is infinitely better than 'permanent death'

from psychotic-depressed-mood-driven suicidal ideation and suicide. In medical and surgical practice, necessary life-saving remedies cannot be all side effect-free.

ECT and psychotic depressive illness have nothing to do with PTSD type 1 and PTSD type 2. But PTSD type 1 and PTSD type 2 can lead to severely depressed moods, severely anxious and angry emotions, and extremes of frustration, all leading to ideas of suicide. Following the Falklands War of 1982, more British soldiers who returned from the war died from PTSD-related suicide than had been killed in the three months of the war itself. Let's not forget that such things happen to too many of those with the unique disorder of PTSD type 1 and or with PTSD type 2, war, or no war. EMDR doesn't cure all people with PTSD type 1—the help of genomics and dedicated genomicists will be needed.

The author of this book, me, had my next sibling, a brother, born when I was eight years old, ensuring that I would grow up to be a narcissist (as any Character Analyst would predict). He remains a life-long friend. I climbed The Matterhorn with my younger girlfriend when I was eighteen, much to the annoyance of the local mountain guides. I left my first love, neurosurgery, in mid-life through boredom, and took to the more philosophical psychiatry, retiring at eighty-two. Sadly, I have had to continue to annoy my peers in my long-continuing search for a better truth about PTSD. Medical science is a tough game.